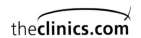
the**clinics.com**

HEMATOLOGY/ ONCOLOGY CLINICS OF NORTH AMERICA

Hairy Cell Leukemia

GUEST EDITOR
Alan Saven, MD

October 2006 • Volume 20 • Number 5

SAUNDERS

An Imprint of Elsevier, Inc.
PHILADELPHIA   LONDON   TORONTO   MONTREAL   SYDNEY   TOKYO

W.B. SAUNDERS COMPANY
A Division of Elsevier Inc.

Elsevier Inc. • 1600 John F. Kennedy Boulevard • Suite 1800 • Philadelphia, Pennsylvania 19103-2899

http://www.hemonc.theclinics.com

HEMATOLOGY/ONCOLOGY CLINICS
OF NORTH AMERICA   Volume 20, Number 5
October 2006   ISSN 0889-8588
Editor: Kerry Holland   ISBN 1-4160-3906-6

The ideas and opinions expressed in *Hematology/Oncology Clinics of North America* do not necessarily reflect those of the Publisher. The Publisher does not assume any responsibility for any injury and/or damage to persons or property arising out of or related to any use of the material contained in this periodical. The reader is advised to check the appropriate medical literature and the product information currently provided by the manufacturer of each drug to be administered to verify the dosage, the method and duration of administration, or contraindications. It is the responsibility of the treating physician or other health care professional, relying on independent experience and knowledge of the patient, to determine drug dosages and the best treatment of the patient. Mention of any product in this issue should not be construed as endorsement by the contributors, editors, or the Publisher of the product or manufacturers' claims.

Hematology/Oncology Clinics (ISSN 0889-8588) is published bimonthly by Elsevier Inc., 360 Park Avenue South, New York, NY 10010-1710. Months of issue are February, April, June, August, October, and December. Business and Editorial Offices: 1600 John F. Kennedy Blvd., Suite 1800, Philadelphia, PA 19103-2899. Customer Service Office: 6277 Sea Harbor Drive, Orlando, FL 32887-4800. Periodicals postage paid at New York, NY and additional mailing offices. Subscription prices are $220.00 per year (US individuals), $330.00 per year (US institutions), $110.00 per year (US students), $250.00 per year (Canadian individuals), $395.00 per year (Canadian institutions), $140.00 per year (Canadian students), $280.00 per year (international individuals), $395.00 per year (international institutions), $140.00 per year (international students). International air speed delivery is included in all *Clinics* subscription prices. All prices are subject to change without notice. **POSTMASTER:** Send address changes to *Hematology/Oncology Clinics of North America*, Elsevier Periodicals Customer Service, 6277 Sea Harbor Drive, Orlando, FL 32887-4800. Customer Service: 1-800-654-2452 (US). From outside of the US, call 1-407-345-4000.

Hematology/Oncology Clinics of North America is covered in *Index Medicus, EMBASE/Excerpta Medica,* and *BIOSIS.*

Printed in the United States of America.

EVIER
INDERS

HEMATOLOGY/ONCOLOGY CLINICS
OF NORTH AMERICA

Hairy Cell Leukemia

GUEST EDITOR

ALAN SAVEN, MD, Head, Division of Hematology/Oncology, Scripps Clinic; and Director, Ida M. and Cecil H. Green Cancer Center, La Jolla, California

CONTRIBUTORS

RAJESH BELANI, MD, Fellow, Division of Hematology/Oncology, Scripps Clinic, La Jolla, California

KELLY J. BETHEL, MD, Hematopathologist, Department of Pathology, Scripps Clinic, La Jolla, California

J.C. CAWLEY, MD, PhD, FRCP, FRCPath, Professor and Head, Department of Haematology, University of Liverpool, Liverpool, United Kingdom

ADI GIDRON, MD, Fellow, Department of Medicine, Division of Hematology/Oncology, Northwestern University Feinberg School of Medicine and The Robert H. Lurie Comprehensive Cancer Center of Northwestern University, Chicago, Illinois

MICHAEL R. GREVER, MD, Chair and Professor, Department of Internal Medicine; Charles A. Doan Chair of Medicine; Co-Program Leader; Experimental Therapeutics for the James Comprehensive Cancer Center, The Ohio State University, Columbus, Ohio

THOMAS M. HABERMANN, MD, Professor, Department of Hematology, Mayo Clinic College of Medicine, Rochester, Minnesota

MARK A. HOFFMAN, MD, Associate Professor of Clinical Medicine, Department of Medicine, Albert Einstein College of Medicine, Bronx; Division of Hematology-Oncology, Department of Medicine, Long Island Jewish Medical Center, New Hyde Park, New York

GUNNAR JULIUSSON, MD, Professor of Hematology, Stem Cell Center, Lund University; Department of Hematology, Lund University Hospital, Lund, Sweden

HAGOP KANTARJIAN, MD, Chair, Department of Leukemia, University of Texas M.D. Anderson Cancer Center, Houston, Texas

ROBERT J. KREITMAN, MD, Chief, Clinical Immunotherapy Section, Laboratory of Molecular Biology, Center for Cancer Research, National Cancer Institute, National Institutes of Health, Bethesda, Maryland

JAN LILIEMARK, MD, Professor, Medical Products Agency, Uppsala, Sweden

ESTELLA MATUTES, MD, PhD, Department of Haemato-Oncology, The Royal Marsden Hospital and Institute of Cancer Research, London, United Kingdom

IRA PASTAN, MD, Chief, Laboratory of Molecular Biology, Center for Cancer Research, National Cancer Institute, National Institutes of Health, Bethesda, Maryland

FARHAD RAVANDI, MD, Assistant Professor, Department of Leukemia, University of Texas M.D. Anderson Cancer Center, Houston, Texas

ALAN SAVEN, MD, Head, Division of Hematology/Oncology, Scripps Clinic; Director, Ida M. and Cecil H. Green Cancer Center, La Jolla, California

ROBERT W. SHARPE, MD, Hematopathologist, Department of Pathology, Scripps Clinic, La Jolla, California

MARTIN S. TALLMAN, MD, Professor, Department of Medicine, Division of Hematology/Oncology, Northwestern University Feinberg School of Medicine and The Robert H. Lurie Comprehensive Cancer Center of Northwestern University, Chicago, Illinois

DEBORAH A. THOMAS, MD, Assistant Professor, Department of Leukemia, University of Texas M.D. Anderson Cancer Center, Houston, Texas

HEMATOLOGY/ONCOLOGY CLINICS
OF NORTH AMERICA

SEVIER
UNDERS

Hairy Cell Leukemia

CONTENTS VOLUME 20 • NUMBER 5 • OCTOBER 2006

In the twenty-first century, gene microarray analysis has confirmed that hairy cells (HCs) are activated late B cells that are related more closely to chronic lymphocytic leukemia and normal memory B cells than to any other B-cell type examined. This approach also revealed the specific expression of several genes that might have pathophysiologic and diagnostic importance. Also, cell-signaling studies have defined the mechanistic basis of several of the distinctive features of HCs; however, such studies have not identified the oncogenic source of these intrinsic signals. Therefore, identification of the oncogenic events that are responsible for the distinctive phenotype of HCs is the biggest remaining challenge in the disease.

The hematopathology of hairy cell leukemia (HCL) is discussed. HCL has distinctive morphologic features that permitted accurate diagnosis even before the development of ancillary methods. In the last several decades flow cytometry and immunohistochemistry have replaced traditional cytochemical and ultrastructural methods for confirming a morphologic impression of HCL. The characteristic morphologic and ancillary findings and the role that they play in discriminating HCL from other neoplasms are described. With the advent of extremely effective chemotherapy for HCL, the evaluation of posttherapy bone marrow biopsies for evidence of residual disease has increased in importance and is discussed. Lastly, the pathology of the variant form of HCL and the relationship of this entity to typical HCL and splenic marginal zone lymphoma are presented.

The cells of hairy cell leukemia and its variant form have a distinct immunophenotype that seems to correspond to that of a mature activated memory B cell. Although the two diseases have similarities in histology and membrane marker expression, such as the selected immunoglobulin heavy-chain expression and the reactivity with certain B-cell activation markers, there are differences in their clinical course, morphology, and immunophenotype. Immunophenotyping is an essential tool for the diagnosis of these two disorders, for monitoring and assessing response to therapy, and for distinguishing them from other B-cell malignancies.

Hairy cell leukemia typically presents in middle-aged men and is characterized by splenomegaly and cytopenias. Hepatomegaly may be present, but usually is not a salient feature. Peripheral adenopathy is uncommon. Other organ manifestations occur but are unusual. Patients are now presenting with a less tumor burden because of earlier diagnosis. Leukocytosis/lymphocytosis should suggest hairy cell leukemia variant. Infectious complications, which were common in the past and the major cause of death, have become rare in the era of purine analog therapy. Whether there is a true increased risk for second malignancies remains controversial.

Hairy cell leukemia (HCL) is an uncommon leukemia. After Hodgkin lymphoma, HCL has been a model for incorporating and understanding the clinical interventions of surgery, chemotherapy, biologic response modifiers, purine nucleoside analogs, and monoclonal antibody therapy. Advances in treatment, all of which were empiric at the time, preceded advancements in understanding the biology of the disease. The history of therapeutic intervention has been characterized by empiric interventions without scientific bench research applied to a disease that did not have good outcomes or therapeutic interventions. Such approaches have changed the natural history of this disease and opened doors for other diseases. Over time, the definitions of response evolved into modern response definitions. This article focuses on treatments of historical interest, observation, splenectomy, and the interferons.

Cladribine is effective therapy for hairy cell leukemia, and there are several ways to achieve the adequate concentrations of the active metabolites in relevant cells, without the need for long-term continuous infusions. This simplifies therapy, although careful control of patients is required during and after treatment in most instances because of the significant activity of the drug on leukemia cells of various types and on lymphoid cells and normal stem cells.

Pentostatin: Impact on Outcome in Hairy Cell Leukemia   1099
Michael R. Grever

Major advances in the management of patients who have hairy cell leukemia have been made following the use of purine nucleoside analogs. Pentostatin and cladribine are equally effective, and have impressive long-term effectiveness. The gradual, but relentless, improvement in the peripheral blood counts enables the outpatient management with pentostatin in most patients. Cladribine affords the convenience of a single course of administration. A direct comparative study with these two agents is unlikely to yield dramatic differences in improvement. Patients still relapse, and the overall survival curves have not reached a plateau, which indicates that cure has not been secured. Future studies should be directed to optimizing the therapy for minimal residual disease as well as clearer definition of supportive care.

Cladribine in Hairy Cell Leukemia   1109
Rajesh Belani and Alan Saven

Cladribine is a purine nucleoside analog that has been applied extensively to the treatment of indolent lymphoid malignancies, especially hairy cell leukemia (HCL). It induces apoptosis of hairy cells, and, thereby, induces prolonged complete remissions in most patients. This article reviews the history, rationale, chemical structure, mechanism of action, clinical activity, and toxicity of cladribine in HCL. Salvage treatments, for relapse after cladribine, also are discussed.

Monoclonal Antibody Therapy for Hairy Cell Leukemia   1125
Deborah A. Thomas, Farhad Ravandi, and Hagop Kantarjian

The use of monoclonal antibody (MoAb) therapy for the treatment of hairy cell leukemia (HCL) offers great promise and potential for improving progression-free survival. Rituximab has activity in previously treated HCL and the ability to eradicate minimal residual disease after 2-chlorodeoxyadenosine given as frontline therapy. Alemtuzumab, epratuzumab, and other candidate MoAb's should be studied in HCL. Appropriate pharmacologic investigations, use of antigen modulation, and assessments of soluble antigen levels should be considered with future clinical trials of MoAb's in HCL to optimize therapeutic strategies.

Immunotoxins in the Treatment of Refractory Hairy Cell Leukemia

Robert J. Kreitman and Ira Pastan

An increasing number of patients who have hairy cell leukemia (HCL) have persistent disease that requires treatment, despite purine analogs, splenectomy, interferon, and rituximab. Many of these patients have been treated successfully with immunotoxins. An immunotoxin contains a protein toxin connected to a cell-binding ligand, such as an antibody. An immunotoxin recognizes the target cell, internalizes, and the toxin translocates to the cytosol where it inhibits protein synthesis enzymatically. Immunotoxins that show activity in HCL contain truncated *Pseudomonas* exotoxin fused to the Fv fragments of anti-CD25 or anti-CD22 monoclonal antibodies. Both agents, termed LMB-2 and BL22, respectively, have been tested in patients who have HCL after failure of purine analogs and other therapies; major responses have been achieved in most patients.

Hairy Cell Leukemia: Towards a Curative Strategy

Adi Gidron and Martin S. Tallman

Although not all patients who have hairy cell leukemia (HCL) require therapy at diagnosis, most eventually will need treatment. Historically, splenectomy and interferon-α resulted in hematologic responses; however, responses tend to be short, as is survival. The introduction of purine analogs dramatically changed the prognosis for most patients who have HCL. It is now considered standard of care to use a purine analog as first-line therapy. This approach results in a high complete remission rate and prolonged disease-free survival. Despite the excellent results with purine analogs, most patients have minimal residual disease detected by sensitive techniques; 30% to 40% of patients eventually relapse and most require further therapy. For patients who have relapsed or refractory disease, monoclonal antibody–based therapies are emerging options.

HEMATOLOGY/ONCOLOGY CLINICS
OF NORTH AMERICA

FORTHCOMING ISSUES

December 2006

Neuro-oncology
Lisa DeAngelis, MD, and Jerome Posner, MD
Guest Editors

February 2007

Inflamation, Hemostasis, and Blood Conservation Strategies
Jerrold H. Levy, MD
Guest Editor

RECENT ISSUES

August 2006

Prostate Cancer
William K. Oh, MD
Guest Editor

June 2006

Immunotherapy of Cancer
Madhav V. Dhodapkar, MD
Guest Editor

April 2006

Radiation Medicine Update for the Practicing Oncologist, Part II
Lisa A. Kachnic, MD, and Charles R. Thomas, Jr. MD
Guest Editors

HEMATOLOGY/ONCOLOGY CLINICS
OF NORTH AMERICA

LSEVIER
AUNDERS

Preface

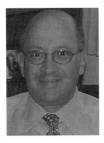

Alan Saven, MD
Guest Editor

airy cell leukemia (HCL) has assumed a level of great medical importance, despite its relative rarity as a chronic lymphoid leukemia. This is
because it is a unique and peculiar clinicopathologic entity that demonstrates unparalleled sensitivity to systemic therapy. Accordingly, it has served
as a model for rational drug development. Although splenectomy regularly
normalizes the disease-associated cytopenias, it is now principally of historic interest because there are three agents approved to treat HCL—namely, interferon, pentostatin, and cladribine. At the Scripps Clinic, we found that single
infusions of cladribine, administered continuously over 7 days, induce response
rates greater than 95%, 85% of which are complete and durable. More recently,
the monoclonal antibody rituximab and the recombinant immunotoxin BL22
have been used in the treatment of this disease. Given the effectiveness of systemic treatments in HCL, it is absolutely mandatory that this entity be recognized when present.

In this issue of the *Hematology/Oncology Clinics of North America*, expert hemato-
pathologists and clinicians, all of whom have been carefully selected, review the
latest pathologic, clinical, and therapeutic advances in this disease and deliber-
ate how this information can be translated into a curative strategy.

Alan Saven, MD
Division of Hematology/Oncology, Scripps Clinic
and Ida M. and Cecil H. Green Cancer Center
10666 North Torrey Pines Road
La Jolla, CA 92037, USA

E-mail address: saven.alan@scrippshealth.org

0889-8588/06/$ – see front matter
doi:10.1016/j.hoc.2006.08.001

Hematol Oncol Clin N Am 20 (2006) 1011–1021

HEMATOLOGY/ONCOLOGY CLINICS
OF NORTH AMERICA

The Pathophysiology of the Hairy Cell

J.C. Cawley, MD, PhD, FRCP, FRCPath

Department of Haematology, University of Liverpool, Third Floor Duncan Building,
Daulby Street, Liverpool L69 3GA, UK

HISTORICAL PERSPECTIVES

Although the disease probably was identified earlier, it was the report of Bouroncle and colleagues [1] in 1958 that firmly established hairy cell leukemia (HCL) as a distinct clinicopathologic entity. This report clearly identified the highly distinctive malignant hairy cells (HCs) that are pathognomonic of the disease. At the time, the nature of these cells was unclear, but their propensity to infiltrate lymphoreticular tissue was recognized and acknowledged in the term "leukemic reticuloendotheliosis" that was used by Bouroncle and colleagues to label the disease.

In 1958, methods for characterizing leukemic cells were limited; therefore, early studies mainly were concerned with the light microscope and ultrastructural appearances of the malignant cells. These studies emphasized the striking and distinctive appearance of the malignant cells, with their prominent and dynamic surface projections or hairs. Therefore, the descriptive and memorable term "hairy cell leukemia" gradually replaced the older term "leukemic reticuloendotheliosis."

In the 1970s, advances in basic immunology and the introduction of some simple methodologies for identifying B and T cells led to numerous attempts to characterize the nature of HCs. Although these early studies were made more difficult by the stickiness of HCs, the general conclusion was that the cells are unusual clonal B cells with no obvious normal counterpart (reviewed in [2]).

The introduction of monoclonal antibodies in the 1980s confirmed this conclusion (reviewed in [3]), as did immunoglobulin rearrangement studies [4]. Furthermore, HCs were found to express antigens that are associated with late B-cell development, as well as with cellular activation (reviewed in [5]). Therefore, since the late 1980s HCL has been regarded as a clonal proliferation of activated late B cells.

In the 1990s, interest moved to aspects of HC behavior that were relevant to clinical disease. For example, work in the author's department was focused on

---

The author's work is supported by the Leukaemia Research Fund (UK).

E-mail address: haem@liverpool.ac.uk

the homing and adhesive properties of HCs relevant to the unusual and distinctive patterns of tissue infiltration in HCL [6–8]. There also was considerable interest in why HCL is so susceptible to interferon and nucleoside therapies [9–11].

In the twenty-first century, gene microarray analysis has confirmed that HCs are activated late B cells that are related more closely to chronic lymphocytic leukemia (CLL) and normal memory B cells than to any other B-cell type examined [12]. This approach also revealed the specific expression of several genes that might have pathophysiologic and diagnostic importance. Also, cell-signaling studies (see later discussion) have defined the mechanistic basis of several of the distinctive features of HCs; however, such studies have not identified the oncogenic source of these intrinsic signals. Therefore, identification of the oncogenic events that are responsible for the distinctive phenotype of HCs is the biggest remaining challenge in the disease.

The pathophysiology of HCs is reviewed in detail using the above historical outline as a basis for presentation of the major features of these unusual and fascinating cells.

CYTOLOGY, CYTOCHEMISTRY, AND ULTRASTRUCTURE

The appearance of HCs in Romanowsky-stained peripheral blood films is now extremely well known (eg, reviewed in [2,3]), and is that of a metabolically active cell with prominent surface projections. It has long been known from phase-contrast microscopic studies of live cells that the surface of HCs is in a constant state of change. Transmission and scanning electron microscopy basically confirmed the conclusion that HCs are highly active cells with a distinctive surface morphology. In addition, transmission electron microscopy revealed the frequent presence of ribosome-lamellar complexes [13]; however, these structures turned out not to be specific for HCs and their functional significance has never been defined.

The finding that HCs specifically express tartrate-resistant acid phosphatase (TRAP; isoenzyme 5) was a triumph of the cytochemistry era [14]. TRAP positivity was, and still is, an important diagnostic aid in the disease, but its pathophysiologic importance remains unclear.

THE PREMONOCLONAL ANTIBODY ERA: HAIRY CELLS AS MATURE B CELLS

The major conclusions at this time were that HCs express light-chain–restricted immunoglobulin (SIg) and receptors for the Fc of IgG (γFcR) at their cell surface. The SIg was unusual in that it consisted of mixed heavy-chain isotopes or of IgG alone [15,16]. The significance of these findings was unclear at the time, but the findings later were confirmed at the molecular level (see later discussion; [17,18]).

The presence of γFcR on HCs is a "monocytoid" feature of the cells [19]; however, this feature of HCs has not been given any further pathophysiologic significance except to say that Fc binding probably was responsible for the propensity of polyclonal antibodies to stick "nonspecifically" to these cells.

THE MONOCLONAL ANTIBODY ERA: HAIRY CELLS AS ACTIVATED MATURE B CELLS

Studies with a range of monoclonal antibodies confirmed the earlier conclusion that HCs are clonal late B cells (Table 1). Thus, HCs express a range of B-cell markers (eg, CD19, CD20, CD22) and their possession of light-chain–restricted SIg was confirmed. Furthermore, although HCs express the plasma-cell antigen PCA1 [20], the malignant cells have little or no propensity to differentiate into antibody-secreting cells. Also, the malignant cells express several antigens (eg, FMC7, CD22, CD25, CD72, CD40L) that are associated with the activation of B cells and other cell types (see Table 1). HCs lack CD23, which is expressed by CLL cells and up-regulated during normal B-cell activation (reviewed in [3]). Therefore, as one might expect, HCs are activated in a different way from CLL cells, which are now believed to be stimulated and selected by (auto)antigen [21]. The search for HC-restricted antigens further supported the notion that the malignant cells are highly activated. Thus, most, if not all, apparently HC-specific reagents (eg, HC-2 and CD103) turned out also to detect antigens that are associated with the activation of certain other lymphoid and nonlymphoid cell types (reviewed in [5]).

FUNCTIONAL STUDIES: ADHESION AND HOMING, CYTOKINES AND SUSCEPTIBILITY TO THERAPY

Adhesion and Homing

The pathology of HCL is distinctive in that the HCs infiltrate the red pulp of the spleen and hepatic sinusoids and portal tracts, but spare lymph nodes (reviewed in [2,3]). Furthermore, HCs modify the infiltrated tissues by causing bone marrow fibrosis and by forming vascular lakes (the so-called "pseudosinuses"), especially in the splenic red pulp. These pathologic features caused the author and colleagues and other investigators to be interested in the

Table 1
Reactivity of hairy cells with antibodies

Presence of B cell antigens	CD19, 20, 22
Absence of germinal center antigens	CD10, BCL-6
Absence of plasma-cell markers	MUM-1, CD138, BLIMP1
Up-regulated activation antigens	FMC-7, CD22, CD25, CD72, CD40L
Down-regulation of antigens often reduced during activation of other cell types	CD21, CD24
HC-'restricted' antigens probably indicative of activation	CD11c, CD68, CD103, HC-2, Cyclin D1, TRAP (often demonstrated cytochemically)
HC-specific antigens of uncertain pathogenetic significance, but of potential diagnostic interest	Annexin A1, CD123 (IL-3R)

mechanisms of these processes. HCs were found consistently to express a range of adhesion receptors (Table 2) [7]. The fact that HCs are highly adherent, and—on some substrates, spontaneously motile cells—indicated that their adhesion/motility receptors are activated constitutively. This conclusion is supported by the fact that HCs interact spontaneously with several extracellular matrix components, including fibronectin (FN) [6], vitronectin (VN) [7], and hyaluronan (HA) [22] (see Table 2 for relevant adhesion receptors).

On FN, HCs firmly adhere and assume a spread morphology [7]. Such spreading on FN in the bone marrow stroma may well be responsible for the distinctive loose packing and "halo" appearance (HCs surrounded by clear areas) that is observed in fixed marrow tissue. The HCs themselves probably are responsible for synthesizing and assembling the FN that is an important constituent of the bone marrow fibrosis of HCL [6]. Regarding the stimulus for FN production, the author and colleagues showed that interaction of HCs (by way of CD44v3) with HA in the bone marrow stimulates autocrine FGF production, which, in turn, stimulates the malignant cells to synthesize FN [22,23]. Because HA is not present in the splenic red pulp or hepatic sinusoids, this probably explains why FN is not present at these sites, despite the presence of extensive HC infiltration.

VN is abundant in spleen and it likely is that interaction of HCs with this protein (by way of $\alpha V \beta 3$) is important in the splenic homing of the malignant

Table 2
Receptors and ligands involved in hairy cell adhesion and homing

Integrins	Adhesion receptors (CD)	Possible functions
$\alpha_4\beta_1$	(49d/29)	Involved in binding to matrix (FN) & accessory cells by way of CD106 (VCAM).
$\alpha_5\beta_1$	(49e/29)	Involved with $\alpha_4\beta_1$ in binding to, and assembly of, FN matrix.
$\alpha_M\beta_2$	(11b/18)	Weakly expressed. Constitutes a monocytic feature of HCs & may be involved in endocytosis.
$\alpha_X\beta_2$	(11c/18)	Diagnostically important. Receptor for several ligands, including ICAM-1 (CD54), but function in HCs unclear.
$\alpha_V\beta_3$	(51/61)	Receptor for vitronectin and PECAM-1 (CD31). Important in HC motility.
$\alpha_E\beta_7$	(103/β_7)	Diagnostically important. Receptor for E cadherin, but function in HCL unclear.
Other adhesion receptors		
CD44		Highly expressed. HC receptor of hyaluronan. Several isoforms expressed (V3, V6). CD44H signals for bFGF production; V3 (heparan sulphate-containing isoform) acts as a coreceptor with FGFR-1 for stimulation of HC FN production by bFGF.
L-selectin	(62L)	Little or no expression. Shed on cell activation.

cells [7]. Regarding the vascular remodelling that is necessary for pseudosinus formation, it is likely that HC interaction with endothelial cells (by way of α4β-to-VCAM) is involved initially [8]. This interaction may be followed by replacement of the endothelial cells by HCs in a process that involves αVβ3-mediated movement of HCs in between and underneath endothelium. The binding partners of αVβ3 during this process could be PECAM on endothelial cells and VN on basement membranes.

Cytokines

Table 3 summarizes what is known about autocrine cytokine production by HCs. Tumor necrosis factor (TNF), interleukin (IL)-6, and granulocyte/macrophage colony-stimulating factor (GM-CSF) promote HC survival/proliferation [24–26], whereas GM-CSF and macrophage colony-stimulating factor affect malignant cell adhesion/motility [27,28]. The role of bFGF in HA-stimulated FN by HCs already was mentioned. Transforming growth factor-β can inhibit normal hematopoiesis and stimulate bone marrow fibroblasts to produce collagen; this cytokine, together with IL-10, also may suppress the immune function of reactive T cells and monocytes [29,30].

HCs also can be influenced by cytokines that are produced by other cells. For example, IL-4 and IL-15, alone or in combination with other growth factors, can stimulate DNA synthesis in the malignant cells [31]. Among B cells, HCs

Table 3
Pathogenetically relevant cytokines produced by hairy cells

Cytokine	Receptors on HCs	Comment
TNF-α	TNFRI and RII present	Involved in HC survival and response to IFN therapy.
IL-6	Present	Production may be induced by TNF. May participate in the proliferative effects of TNF.
IL-10	Not studied	Suppresses TH1 cytokine production.
GM-CSF	Receptor present	Prolongs the survival of HCs & inhibits their motility.
M-CSF	Receptor present	Stimulates chemokinesis & chemotaxis of HCs.
bFGF	FGFR1 and CD44v3 coreceptor present	Involved in FN production by HA-adherent HCs. May stimulate increased angiogenesis in HCL BM.
TGFβ	Not studied	Elevated in HCL serum and BM. May be involved in suppression of the production & function of normal hematologic cells, & stimulates BM fibroblasts to produce the collagen component of reticulin fibrosis.
IFNα	Receptor present	Induces HC apoptosis in the absence of cell adhesion and may induce autocrine TNF production.

express receptors that are relatively specific for IL-2 (CD25) [4] and IL-3 (CD123) [32], and detection of these receptors has diagnostic importance; however, no functional effects of either interleukin on HCs have been demonstrated.

The Susceptibility of Hairy Cells to Interferon and Nucleoside

Among all hemic malignancies, HCL is unusually sensitive to α–interferon and nucleosides (deoxycoformycin, chlorodeoxyadenosine, fludarabine). Therefore, the mechanisms that are involved in this high and relatively specific sensitivity were/are of considerable interest.

Regarding the sensitivity of HCs to interferon, it seems likely that autocrine TNF plays a central role. The malignant cells produce large amounts of TNF and possess TNF receptors 1 and 2 [9–11]. Autocrine TNF-α increases cell survival [33], but in the presence of α-interferon this prosurvival effect is converted to a proapoptotic one [11]. This killing is brought about by interferon-induced suppression of the production of inhibitors of apoptosis (IAPs), which is regulated by the nuclear factor κB (NFκB)-dependent arm of TNF signaling. HC adhesion to VN and FN stimulates IAP production that is not inhibited by α-interferon [11]. Therefore, such adhesion can provide relative protection of HCs from interferon-induced, TNF-mediated killing [11]. This may explain why, during interferon therapy, HCs persist in the spleen and bone marrow long after they have been cleared from the blood.

Much is known about how nucleosides induce apoptosis in resting lymphocytes (reviewed in [34]); however, it remains unclear why HCs are so sensitive to the apoptotic effects of this class of reagents.

TWENTY-FIRST CENTURY: GENE EXPRESSION PROFILING, IGVH MUTATIONAL ANALYSIS, AND CYTOGENETIC AND CELL-SIGNALING STUDIES

Gene Expression Profiling: Hairy Cells are Related to Memory Cells

DNA microarray analysis demonstrated that HCL cases display a largely homogenous phenotype that is distinct from that of other B-cell malignancies, and that HCs more resemble memory B cells than any of the other B-cell types examined [12]. This seems a convenient point to consider surface CD27, a marker of normal memory B cells. Although the microarray study of Basso and colleagues [12] found that CD27 was present in most of the HCL samples at the message level, a recent study failed to detect CD27 protein in all cases of HCL studied [35]. The significance of this discrepancy is not clear. In addition to showing that HCs are related to memory cells, the microarray analysis showed that HCs specifically express several genes and differ from memory cells in their expression of genes for cytokines/chemokines and adhesion receptors. Eighty-two genes were overexpressed specifically, whereas only 7 were down-regulated; some of these where overexpression was validated at the protein level are listed in Table 4. In particular, the microarray analysis identified a new possible diagnostic marker, annexin A1 [36], and defined several genes that are involved in adhesion/motility/tissue invasion that had not been linked

Table 4
Some genes of potential pathogenetic importance specifically up-or down-regulated in hairy cells

Gene	Possible significance
Up-regulated	
Annexin A1 ⎱ IL-3Rα ⎰	Pathogenetic significance unclear, but specific expression of diagnostic value.
Cyclin D	Overexpression confined to HCL and mantle cell lymphoma, but functional significance unclear.
GAS7 ⎱ EPB4.IL2 ⎰	Interact with actin; probably important in maintaining HC shape.
β actin	Essential for maintaining HC shape and motility.
Plexin C1	Involved in integrin-mediated motility.
TIMP-1 ⎱ TIMP-4 ⎰	Inhibit MMPs; may inhibit tissue invasion by HCs.
bFGF ⎱ FGFR1 ⎰	Implicated in the production of FN by HCs; relevant to BM fibrosis.
Synaptotagmin1	Involved in Ca^{2+} signaling for exocytosis.
Down-regulated[a]	
CXCR5	Receptor for CXCL13 (BLC or BCA-1) chemokine necessary for follicular homing; down-regulation may be relevant to absence of lymph nodes in HCL.
TRAF5	Involved in signal transduction by TNF-type receptors.

[a]Not confirmed at protein level.

previously with these processes in HCs. Also, the analysis confirmed the probable importance of autocrine bFGF in the bone marrow fibrosis of the disease.

IgVH Mutational Analysis: Hairy Cells Usually Have Hypermutated VH Genes

In most cases of HCL, the malignant cells have mutated VH genes with low levels of intraclonal variability [17,18,36,38]; this is compatible with the gene array data that suggest that HCs are memory cells. Furthermore, HCs express activation-induced cytidine deaminase [18], a molecule that is essential for somatic mutation and isotope switching; however, in up to approximately 20% of cases, no significant VH mutation is observed [18]. What this means in relation to the developmental stage of such clones is not clear. Regarding VH gene family usage, a recent report found VH 3-30 in 6 of 32 (19%) patients studied. The investigators interpreted this finding as indicating involvement of antigenic selection in the development of HCL [37].

Regarding the expression of multiple heavy-chain isotopes, this phenomenon has been studied in some detail [17,18]. First of all, VH sequencing confirmed earlier studies at the protein level that indicated that single cells can express multiple heavy-chain isotypes simultaneously [17,18]. Normally, isotype-switching recombination is brought about by deletional recombination, which generates extrachromosomal circular DNA. Forconi and colleagues [18] found no evidence of such switch circles in HCs that expressed multiple heavy-chain isotypes. They interpreted this as indicating that multiple transcripts are being generated at the RNA level, and that such cells are arrested at a point of isotype switching before deletional recombination. In contrast, HCs that express a single heavy-chain isotype have achieved deletional isotype switching [39].

Cytogenetics: Hairy Cells Have No Consistent or Specific Abnormalities

Although many karyotypic abnormalities have been described in HCL, none are specific and none are found consistently in the disease. As pointed out by Basso and colleagues [12], HCs, unlike other malignant B cells apart from CLL lymphocytes, typically lack reciprocal balanced chromosomal transloca-tions. Because these translocations are generated during VDJ recombination, class switching, and somatic hypermutation, their absence supports the micro-array data that suggest that HCL and CLL are malignancies of mature mem-ory B cells in which these processes have been switched off [12,40,41].

Regarding cytogenetic abnormalities reported in HCL, the most frequent are gains of parts of chromosome 5 ($\sim$20%) [42,43] or losses of the long arm of chromosome 7 ($\sim$10%) [43]. A recent comparative expressed sequence hybrid-ization analysis found several under- or overexpressed regions that contain many of the genes that are expressed differentially in gene microarray analysis [44]; however, cytogenetic studies have not provided firm clues concerning pos-sible oncogenic events in HCL. Furthermore, considering the apparent homo-geneity of the disease and the fact that a given chromosome abnormality is present in only a minority of cases, it seems unlikely that any of the identified karyotypic abnormalities are of primary importance in the malignant transfor-mation of HCs.

Cell Signaling Studies: Specific Activation Features of Hairy Cells Confirmed

Given the highly activated nature of HCs, identification of the signaling basis of this activation has been of obvious interest. Also, there is the hope that identi-fication of the upstream origin of constitutive signals may point to the nature of the underlying oncogenic events in the disease.

It was shown early on that Src [45] and phosphorylated CD20/Ca^{2+}/calmod-ulin kinase II [46–48] are involved in the constitutive activation of HCs. Sub-sequently, the author and colleagues found that ERK is activated constitutively in HCs, and that Src and a PKC are involved in this mitogen-ac-tivated protein kinase stimulation. Furthermore, this constitutively active ERK is important in HC survival [49]. Constitutively active Src also is implicated in the activation of RhoGTPases, which, in turn, are responsible for the active cy-toskeleton that is necessary for the distinctive surface morphology of HCs [50]. Recently, the author and colleagues found that HCs specifically express a Ca^{2+}-dependent, but Rac1- and PKC-independent, oxidase (NOX5) [51]. The NOX5 colocalized with, and negatively regulated, the protein tyrosine phosphatase, SHP-1 [51], and, thereby, contributed to the constitutive protein tyrosine phosphorylation that is found in HCs [52].

In conclusion, signaling studies have shed light on the signals that are necessary for cell survival (PKCs, Src, ERK), for cytoskeletal activation (RhoGTPases, Src), for oxidant production and maintenance of protein tyrosine phosphorylation (Ca, NOX5), and for susceptibility to α-interferon (Ca^{2+}, TNF, NFκB, IAPs). These signals have not been traced to their oncogenic origins, however.

SUMMARY

- HCs are clonal late B cells that are related to memory cells and display specific features of activation.
- Many of the distinctive features of HCs (eg, morphology, TRAP) are related to this specific activation.
- Many of the distinctive histologic features of HCL can be related to constitutive production of cytokines (eg, FGF, fibrosis) and to the expression/activation of adhesion receptors (eg, $\alpha_4\beta_1$, $\alpha_5\beta_1$ and $\alpha_v\beta_3$ integrins, CD44v3).
- HCs usually have mutated IgVH genes and have no consistent or specific chromosome abnormalities (5q additions and 7q deletions in a minority).
- The signals that are responsible for several of the phenotypic features of HCs have been identified, but the nature of the underlying oncogenic events remains unknown.

References

[1] Bouroncle BA, Wiseman BK, Doan CA. Leukemic reticuloendotheliosis. Blood 1958;13(7): 609–30.

[2] Cawley JC, Burns GF, Hayhoe FGJ. In: Hairy-cell leukaemia. Berlin: Springer-Verlag; 1980. p. 60–2.

[3] Burthem J, Cawley JC. In: Hairy-cell leukaemia. Berlin: Springer-Verlag; 1996. p. 66–70.

[4] Korsemeyer SJ, Greene WC, Cossman J. Rearrangement and expression of immunoglobulin genes and expression of TAC antigen in hairy cell leukaemia. Proc Natl Acad Sci U S A 1983;80(14):4522–6.

[5] Zuzel M, Cawley JC. The biology of hairy cells. Best Pract Res Clin Haematol 2003;16(1): 1–13.

[6] Burthem J, Cawley JC. The bone marrow fibrosis of hairy cell leukemia is caused by the synthesis and assembly of a fibronectin matrix by the hairy cells. Blood 1994;83(2): 497–504.

[7] Burthem J, Baker PK, Hunt JA, et al. Hairy cell interactions with extracellular matrix: expression of specific integrin receptors and their role in the cell's response to specific adhesive proteins. Blood 1994;84(3):873–82.

[8] Vincent AM, Burthem J, Brew R, et al. Endothelial interactions of hairy cells: the importance of alpha4beta1 in the unusual tissue distribution of the disorder. Blood 1996;88(10): 3945–52.

[9] Billard C, Sigaux F, Wietzerbin J. IFN-α in vivo enhances tumor necrosis factor receptor levels on hairy cells. J Immunol 1990;145(6):1713–8.

[10] Jansen JH, Wientjens GJ, Willemze R, et al. Production of tumour necrosis factor-α by normal and malignant B lymphocytes in response to interferon-α, interferon-γ and interleukin-4. Leukemia 1992;6(2):116–9.

[11] Baker PK, Pettitt AR, Slupsky JR, et al. Response of hairy cells to IFN-α involves induction of apoptosis through autocrine TNF-α and protection by adhesion. Blood 2002;100(2): 647–53.

[12] Basso K, Liso A, Tiacci E, et al. Gene expression profiling of hairy cell leukemia reveals a phenotype related to memory B cells with altered expression of chemokine and adhesion receptors. J Exp Med 2004;199(1):59–68.

[13] Katayama I, Li CY, Yam LT. Ultrastructural characteristics of the 'hairy cells' of leukemic reticuloendotheliosis. Am J Pathol 1972;67(2):361–70.

[14] Yam LT, Li CY, Lam KW. Tartrate-resistant acid phosphatase isoenzyme in the reticulum cells of leukemic reticuloendotheliosis. N Engl J Med 1971;284(7):357–60.

[15] Burns GF, Cawley JC, Worman CP, et al. Multiple hairy chain isotypes on the surface of the cells of hairy-cell leukaemia. Blood 1978;52(6):1132–47.

[16] Jansen J, Schuit HRE, Meijer JLM, et al. Cell markers in hairy cell leukemia studied in cells from 51 patients. Blood 1982;59(1):52–60.

[17] Forconi F, Sahota SS, Raspadori D, et al. Tumor cells of hairy cell leukemia express multiple clonally related immunoglobulin isotypes via RNA splicing. Blood 2001;98(4): 1774–81.

[18] Forconi F, Sahota SS, Raspadori D, et al. Hairy cell leukemia: at the crossroad of somatic mutation and isotype switch. Blood 2004;104(10):3312–7.

[19] Burns GF, Cawley JC. A re-examination of the alleged monocytic features of hairy-cell leukemia. Scand J Haematol 1979;22(5):386–96.

[20] Anderson KC, Boyd AW, Fisher DC, et al. Hairy cell leukemia: a tumour of pre-plasma cells. Blood 1985;65(3):620–9.

[21] Chiorazzi N, Ferrarini M. B cell chronic lymphocytic leukemia: lessons learned from studies of the B cell antigen receptor. Annu Rev Immunol 2003;21:841–94.

[22] Aziz KA, Till KJ, Zuzel M, et al. Involvement of CD44-hyaluronan interaction in malignant cell homing and fibronectin synthesis in hairy cell leukemia. Blood 2000;96(9):3161–7.

[23] Aziz KA, Till KJ, Chen H, et al. The role of autocrine FGF-2 in the distinctive bone marrow fibrosis of hairy-cell leukemia (HCL). Blood 2003;102(3):1051–6.

[24] Schiller JH, Bittner G, Spriggs DR. Tumour necrosis factor, but not other hematopoietic growth factors, prolongs the survival of hairy cell leukaemia cells. Leuk Res 1992;16(4):337–46.

[25] Barut B, Chauhan D, Uchiyama H, et al. Interleukin-6 functions as an intracellular growth factor in hairy cell leukemia in vitro. J Clin Invest 1993;92(5):2346–52.

[26] Harris RJ, Pettitt AR, Schmutz C, et al. Granulocyte-macrophage colony stimulating factor as an autocrine survival factor of mature normal and malignant B lymphocytes. J Immunol 2000;164(7):3887–93.

[27] Till KJ, Burthem J, Lopez A, et al. Granulocyte-macrophage colony stimulating factor receptor: stage-specific expression and function on late B cells. Blood 1996;88(2):479–86.

[28] Burthem J, Baker PK, Hunt JA, et al. The function of c-fms in hairy-cell leukemia: macrophage colony stimulating factor stimulates hairy-cell movement. Blood 1994;83(5):1381–9.

[29] Beck C, Schreiber H, Rowley D. Role of TGF-beta in immune-evasion of cancer. Microsc Res Tech 2001;52(4):387–95.

[30] Prud'homme GJ, Piccirillo CA. The inhibitory effects of transforming growth factor -beta-1 (TGF-beta1) in autoimmune diseases. J Autoimmun 2000;14(1):23–42.

[31] Barut BA, Cochran MK, O'Hara C, et al. Response patterns of hairy cell leukemia to B-cell mitogens and growth factors. Blood 1990;76(10):2091–7.

[32] Del Guidice I, Matutes E, Morilla R, et al. The diagnostic value of CD123 in B-cell disorders with hairy or villous lymphocytes. Haematologica 2004;89(3):303–8.

[33] Cordingley FT, Bianchi A, Hoffbrand AV, et al. Tumour necrosis factor as an autocrine tumour growth factor for chronic B-cell malignancies. Lancet 1988;1(8592):969–71.

[34] Carson DA, Leoni LM. Hairy-cell leukaemia as a model for drug development. Best Pract Res Clin Haematol 2003;16(1):83–9.

[35] Forconi F, Raspadori D, Lenoci M, et al. Absence of surface CD27 distinguishes hairy cell leukemia from other leukemic B-cell malignancies. Haematologica 2005;90(2):266–8.

[36] Falini B, Tiacci E, Liso A, et al. Simple diagnostic assay for hairy cell leukaemia by immuno-cytochemical detection of annexin A1 (ANXA1). Lancet 2004;363(9424):1869–70.

[37] Thorsélius M, Walsh SH, Thunberg U, et al. Heterogeneous somatic hypermutation status confounds the cell of origin in hairy cell leukemia. Leuk Res 2005;29(2):153–8.

[38] Maloum K, Magnac C, Azgui Z, et al. VH gene expression in hairy cell leukaemia. Br J Haematol 1998;101(1):171–8.

[39] Vaandrager JW, Schuuring E, Kluin-Nelemans HC, et al. DNA filter fluorescence in situ hybridization analysis of immunoglobulin class switching in B-cell neoplasia; aberrant CH gene arrangements in follicle centre-cell lymphoma. Blood 1998;92(8):2871–8.

[40] Klein U, Tu Y, Stolovitzki GA, et al. Gene expression profiling of B cell chronic lymphocytic leukemia reveals a homogeneous phenotype related to memory cells. J Exp Med 2001; 194(11):1625–38.

[41] Rosenwald A, Alizadeh AA, Widhopf G, et al. Relation of gene expression phenotype to immunoglobulin mutation genotype in B cell chronic lymphocytic leukemia. J Exp Med 2001;194(11):1639–47.

[42] Wu X, Ivanova G, Merup M, et al. Molecular analysis of the human chromosome 5q13.3 region in patients with hairy cell leukemia and identification of tumour suppressor gene candidates. Genomics 1999;60(2):161–71.

[43] Anderson CL, Gruszka-Westwood A, Ostergaard M, et al. A marrow deletion of 7q is common to HCL and SMZL, but not CLL. Eur J Haematol 2004;72(6):390–402.

[44] Vanhentenrijk V, De Wolf-Peeters C, Wlodarska I. Comparative expressed sequence hybridization studies of hairy-cell leukaemia show uniform expression profile and imprint of spleen signature. Blood 2004;104(1):250–5.

[45] Lynch SA, Brugge JS, Fromowitz F, et al. Increased expression of the Src proto-oncogene in hairy cell leukemia and a subgroup of B-cell lymphomas. Leukemia 1993;7(9): 1416–22.

[46] Genot E, Valentine MA, Degos L, et al. Hyperphosphorylation of CD20 in hairy cells. Alteration by low molecular weight B cell growth factor and IFN-alpha. J Immunol 1991;146(3): 870–8.

[47] Genot E, Bismuth G, Degos L, et al. Interferon-alpha downregulates the abnormal intracytoplasmic free calcium concentration of tumor cells in hairy cell leukemia. Blood 1992;80(8): 2060–5.

[48] Genot E, Meier KE, Licciardi KA, et al. Phosphorylation of CD20 in cells from hairy cell leukemia line. Evidence for involvement of calcium/calmodulin-dependent protein kinase II. J Immunol 1993;151(1):71–82.

[49] Kamiguti AS, Harris RJ, Slupsky JR, et al. Regulation of hairy-cell survival through constitutive activation of mitogen-activated protein kinase pathways. Oncogene 2003;22(15): 2272–84.

[50] Zhang X, Machii T, Matsumara I, et al. Constitutively activated Rho guanosine triphosphatases regulate the growth and morphology of hairy cell leukemia cells. Int J Hematol 2003;77(3):263–73.

[51] Kamiguti AS, Serrander L, Lin K, et al. Expression and activity of NOX5 in the circulating malignant B cells of hairy cell leukemia. J Immunol 2005;175(12):8424–30.

[52] Cawley JC, Zuzel M, Caligaris-Cappio F. Biology of the hairy cell. In: Tallman MS, Polliack A, editors. Hairy cell leukemia. Amsterdam: Harwood Academic Publishers; 2000. p. 9–18.

Hematol Oncol Clin N Am 20 (2006) 1023–1049

HEMATOLOGY/ONCOLOGY CLINICS
OF NORTH AMERICA

Hairy Cell Leukemia: Diagnostic Pathology

Robert W. Sharpe, MD*, Kelly J. Bethel, MD

Department of Pathology, Scripps Clinic, 10666 North Torrey Pines Road, La Jolla, CA 92037, USA

Hairy cell leukemia (HCL) is a low-grade B-cell lymphoproliferative disorder with distinctive morphologic, cytochemical, and immunologic characteristics that permit accurate diagnosis and distinction from other disorders in nearly all cases, often with a limited diagnostic evaluation. In a few patients, atypical features, either clinical or morphologic, require a more complete battery of testing to establish a diagnosis of HCL. The diagnostic criteria of this disorder, as well as other low-grade B-cell lymphoproliferations, have been refined over the past several decades, bringing into focus another far less common lymphoproliferative process that has been termed the variant form of HCL (HCL-V). The pathology of these two disorders, with particular emphasis on a practical approach to the diagnostic hematopathology of HCL, is the topic of this article.

THE HAIRY CELL
Cytology
"Accurate diagnosis of this disease rests upon the recognition of the...cells in blood, bone marrow, or spleen. Morphologic observation of these pathognomonic cells is more art than science..." [1]. This trenchant observation of Yam and colleagues is as relevant today as when it was written in 1972 and emphasizes that, despite the ever-growing battery of ancillary studies to assist the hematopathologist, the identification of cytologically characteristic cells remains the diagnostic *sine qua non* of HCL [2–5]. As such, it is critical to obtain air-dried cytologic material for Wright's and cytochemical stains. Suitable preparations include smears of the peripheral blood or bone marrow and touch preparations of biopsy samples. The routine preparation of bone marrow core biopsy touch preparations should be a standard component of all bone marrow biopsies, but especially so in patients with inaspirable marrow.

In Wright-stained preparations, the hairy cell is 1.5 to 2 times the size of a mature lymphocyte and the nucleus occupies one half to two thirds of the cell's

*Corresponding author. E-mail address: sharpe.robert@scrippshealth.org (R.W. Sharpe).

0889-8588/06/$ – see front matter
doi:10.1016/j.hoc.2006.06.010

area. HCL tends to be a disease of monotonous cells with respect to cytologic characteristics and size. Hence, although there may be a moderate degree of cell size variation between patients, an individual patient usually displays a remarkably homogeneous population of hairy cells (Fig. 1).

The nuclei can have several configurations, including round, oval, spindled, reniform, horseshoe-shaped, and bilobed. Although the hairy cells in an individual vary in nuclear contours, most patients have a preponderant nuclear shape, most commonly oval. Despite variation in nuclear contour, there are several consistent nuclear characteristics of HCL that assist greatly in recognition. Most important, the nuclear membrane is nearly always smooth, imparting a distinct demarcation from the surrounding cytoplasm and lacking the fine surface irregularities that typify many other lymphoproliferative disorders. As well, the nuclear membrane usually appears thickened. The chromatin of HCL

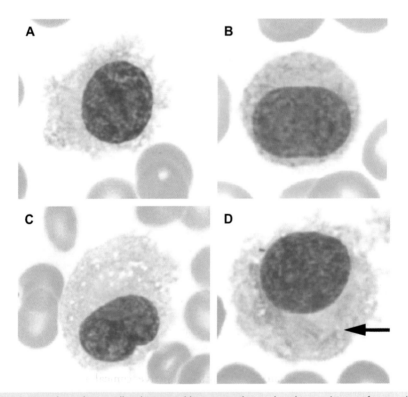

Fig. 1. (A) Classic hairy cell with a smoothly contoured, round nucleus and a rim of textured cytoplasm with circumferential hairlike projections. Peripheral blood (Wright's stain, original magnification ×100). (B) Hairy cells often have an oval nuclear contour and a single small nucleolus. Peripheral blood (Wright's stain, original magnification ×100). (C) The nuclei of hairy cells frequently are reniform to lobated. The cytoplasm has a textured, flocculent appearance. Peripheral blood (Wright's stain, original magnification ×100). (D) Hairy cell with a ribosome-lamella complex (*arrow*). Peripheral blood (Wright's stain, original magnification ×100).

has a partially condensed appearance that is intermediate between a mature lymphocyte and a blast. Additionally, the chromatin has a uniform granular appearance in contrast to the irregularly clumped chromatin of other disorders, particularly B-cell chronic lymphocytic leukemia (B-CLL) and splenic marginal zone lymphoma (SMZL). Hairy cells have no evident nucleoli or a single nucleolus. Infrequently, cells with two nucleoli are present. Generally, patients demonstrate a predominance of nucleolated or nonnucleolated cells. The nucleoli are nearly always small, round, and without irregularities in contour.

The cytoplasm of the hairy cell is distinctive. Although the term "hairy cell" derives from supravital preparations that optimally display the unique topology of these cells, air-dried preparations usually reveal occasional cells with a characteristic corona of cytoplasmic hairlike projections. More commonly, the hairy cell has an indistinct cytoplasmic border that is described as serrated, frayed, or wind-blown. In bone marrow aspirate or touch preparations, there often are many bare nuclei, devoid of cytoplasm. The character of the cytoplasm also is useful in identification. The cytoplasm stains pale gray-blue and because of the frayed margins and pale staining it often merges imperceptibly with the unstained background of the blood smear. The cytoplasm has a textured, flocculent appearance imparted by the presence of irregularly distributed areas of more intense staining. In occasional cases, gray-blue circular and rod-shaped structures, which represent ribosome-lamella complexes, are visible in the cytoplasm (see "Ultrastructural findings" below). These structures have an appearance that is similar in shape and tincture to Dohle bodies that are present in neutrophils of reactive processes and May-Hegglin anomaly [6], while lacking the azurophilic staining and crystalline appearance of Auer rods. The central pale zone of the ribosome-lamella complex is observed occasionally (see Fig. 1D).

Within the spectrum of HCL are occasional patients who manifest unusual cytologic features, most commonly a predominance of hairy cells with horseshoe, spindle, or lobated nuclear contours (Fig. 2) [7,8]. As well, there are rare examples of HCL that are characterized by cells that are comparable in size to large cell lymphoma [9]. Despite the variation in nuclear contour or cell size, the hairy cells demonstrate otherwise typical cytologic features, particularly in the character of chromatin and cytoplasm. HCL patients who have these unusual cytologic features demonstrate clinical, morphologic, and immunophenotypic characteristics that are otherwise typical. Hence, it is important to distinguish HCL with atypical cytologic features, from the variant form of HCL (HCL-V), a separate entity with distinctive clinical and morphologic characteristics.

HCL has an extremely low proliferative rate that manifests cytologically as a virtual absence of transformed cells. Hence, although a variable number of prolymphocytes and paraimmunoblasts typify the cytologic findings of B-CLL and a small percentage of immunoblasts or centroblast-like cells are present in SMZL, transformed cells with prominent nucleoli and increased cytoplasmic basophilia are present rarely in HCL. This characteristic is useful in the cytologic

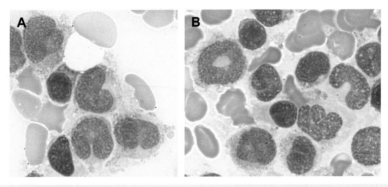

Fig. 2. (A) This is a cytologically unusual variant of otherwise typical HCL. The cells are large and have horseshoe-shaped and lobated nuclei. Peripheral blood (Wright's stain, original magnification ×100). (B) The same patient as in (A) had many cells with a cytoplasmic nuclear inclusion imparting a donutlike appearance. This patient survived for 15 years following a single course of 2-Chlorodeoxyadenosine (2-CdA) without recurrent HCL. Peripheral blood (Wright's stain, original magnification ×100).

differential diagnosis of HCL from other indolent B-cell lymphoproliferative processes.

Ultrastructural Findings

A plethora of publications during the 1970s was devoted to the ultrastructural characteristics of the hairy cell [10–13]. The distinctive hairlike cytoplasmic projections are demonstrable readily by transmission electron microscopy as are nuclear characteristics of peripherally arrayed heterochromatin and the inconsistent presence of a small nucleolus. The most distinctive ultrastructural finding is the ribosome-lamella complex, which is composed of a tubular concentric array of alternating lamellae and free-lying ribosomes with a central zone devoid of either of these components. These structures, which are present in about half of patients who have HCL, often exceed 1 μm in diameter and 3 μm in length. Hence, they can be resolved easily with light microscopy as Dohle body–like cytoplasmic structures (see Fig. 1D) [6]. Ribosome-lamella complexes are not unique to HCL, but are present only infrequently in other low-grade lymphoproliferative disorders. Hence, the on-going diagnostic usefulness of the light microscopic identification of this structure is the predominant enduring legacy to the pathology of HCL from the heyday of diagnostic electron microscopy.

Tartrate-Resistant Acid Phosphatase

A critical cytochemical feature of the hairy cell is the expression of isoenzyme 5 of acid phosphatase that is uniquely resistant to treatment with tartaric acid. This characteristic was exploited in the 1970s by the development of cytochemical stains that permitted the identification of tartrate-resistant acid phosphatase (TRAP) activity of cells in cytologic preparations [14]. Virtually all cases of

HCL show expression of TRAP. In contrast, TRAP positivity is demonstrable in only a small percentage of patients with other lymphoproliferative disorders including B-CLL, Sezary syndrome, T-cell prolymphocytic leukemia, and Human T-cell lymphotrophic virus-1 (HTLV-1)–related T-cell leukemia/lymphoma, diseases that are included rarely in the differential diagnosis of HCL [15,16]. Moreover, the bright expression of TRAP is almost exclusive to HCL. TRAP was the principal study that was used during the last decades of the twentieth century to buttress a morphologic diagnosis of HCL. Although immunophenotypic analysis has supplanted the TRAP stain in many centers over the past decade, the procedure retains significant usefulness in the diagnosis of HCL, and seems to have superior specificity to immunohistochemical TRAP stains (see later discussion). Acid phosphatase stains are particularly useful when fresh tissue is not available for phenotypic analysis or in the evaluation of borderline processes with ambiguous morphologic or immunophenotypic features.

A long discussion of TRAP staining is precluded by its fading usefulness under siege by the on-going introduction of useful flow cytometric and immunohistochemical markers; however, a few comments regarding the interpretation of these stains are relevant to this discussion.

Acid phosphatase stains are technically challenging, and it is critical to confirm their validity, particularly if the stains are used infrequently. Staining for acid phosphatase activity without tartrate treatment always should be performed and reviewed to ensure that there is appropriate staining of normal cells, particularly monocytes and lymphocytes. In the tartrate-treated slides, it is critical to confirm that acid phosphatase activity has been extinguished from these normal cells. Conversely, when TRAP stains are negative, it is generally impractical to exclude a false negative study, as positive control slides rarely are available because of the lability of TRAP activity in air-dried preparations.

A second critical consideration is the definition of a positive TRAP stain. Hairy cells often are heterogeneous in the expression of TRAP with many negative cells. Interpretation of a stain as positive is based predominantly on the intensity of the reaction in individual cells, rather than the number of positive cells. Only a few brightly positive mononuclear cells with cytologic features of HCL are required for a positive study (Fig. 3).

Antigen Expression

General comments

Despite the nostalgic attractiveness of electron microscopy and cytochemical stains, reality beckons recognition that these methodologies have been supplanted by antibody-mediated identification of expressed antigens as the ancillary method of choice in the confirmation of a morphologic diagnosis of HCL. Immunophenotypic characterization by flow cytometry and immunohistochemical staining of tissue sections are the predominant ancillary methods that are employed in the diagnosis of HCL in the twenty-first century. These

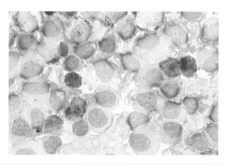

Fig. 3. TRAP stain of HCL showing bright granular cytoplasmic positivity in a minority of the leukemic cells. Bone marrow aspirate (tartrate-treated acid phosphatase stain, original magnification ×100).

methodologies are complementary, and access to both is warranted for the optimal diagnosis and assessment of HCL.

The advantages of flow cytometry include

Simultaneous multi-parameter assessment for the expression of multiple antigens as well as light scattering characteristics. The capacity to evaluate cells for a profile of three to six (and more) antigens provides a high degree of specificity and sensitivity.

Superior sensitivity relative to immunohistochemistry for detecting dim expression of surface antigens

Larger library of antigens that can be assessed

Use of fresh, unfixed tissue, which reduces the number of preanalytical variables that adversely impact tissue immunoreactivity

Unfortunately, the requirement for fresh tissue is also the chief disadvantage of flow cytometry, because HCL often presents with a dearth of circulating hairy cells and "dry tap" bone marrow aspiration that preclude this analysis unless an unfixed portion of the bone marrow core biopsy is available. Another liability is the inability to correlate cytologic findings and antigen expression patterns directly. Finally, assessment for expression of cytoplasmic antigens by flow cytometry often is technically challenging.

The chief strengths of immunohistochemical stains are

Direct visualization of positive cells

Use of readily available fixed and embedded tissue

Meaningful quantification of marrow involvement by HCL

Superior assessment of antigens that are expressed only in the cytoplasm or nucleus

The inability to assess for expression of multiple antigens on a single slide and insensitivity relative to flow cytometry in the detection of dim surface antigen expression are the chief drawbacks of immunohistochemistry. As well, the deleterious effects of preanalytical specimen processing, including fixation and decalcification, must be considered, particularly when assessing the significance of negative studies.

Flow cytometry

Immunophenotypic analysis by flow cytometry is addressed extensively elsewhere in this issue and is summarized briefly here. Hairy cells have a distinctive antigen expression profile that can confirm a morphologic impression of HCL. Nevertheless, flow cytometry was used infrequently in the clinical diagnosis of HCL until the 1990s. Since that time, the development of multi-parameter flow cytometry and antibodies of high specificity have permitted the reliable identification of hairy cells, even when they compose less than 0.5% of analyzed cells [17]. Because small populations of circulating hairy cells are present in nearly all untreated patients who have HCL, these developments have established a primary role for immunophenotypic analysis in the diagnosis of HCL.

When CD45 expression and side scatter characteristics are used in the gating of analyzed cells, the distinctive surface irregularities of hairy cells impart side scatter characteristics that frequently locate them within the monocyte gate [18]. At the same time, the monocyte gate in HCL usually is conspicuously devoid of actual monocytes. The characteristic finding of monoclonal B lymphocytes within the monocyte gate is used in many laboratories as a trigger for assessment of HCL-specific antigens.

The typical phenotypic profile of HCL is characterized by the expression of B-cell markers with bright expression of CD20 and CD22. Hairy cells commonly express bright monotypic surface immunoglobulin although occasional cases are surface immunoglobulin negative. Hairy cells almost never express CD5, whereas about 10% of cases show expression of CD10 [19].

Three markers are of particular usefulness in the phenotypic characterization of HCL. Hairy cells show consistent bright expression of CD11c and are almost always positive for CD103 and CD25 [20]. Expression of these markers is not exclusive to HCL. CD11c is expressed commonly in B-CLL and SMZL; however, the intensity of expression of CD11c in HCL is 30-fold greater than in B-CLL and SMZL. Hence, the bright expression of this antigen has a high degree of specificity for HCL. Similarly, CD25 is expressed in other types of B-cell lymphoproliferative disorders, including nearly half of B-CLL. The expression of CD25 tends to be brighter in HCL than in other lymphoproliferative diseases, but with significant overlap in intensity that limits the specificity of this marker. Nevertheless, CD25 is expressed consistently in hairy cells, and the absence of expression of this antigen in a lymphoproliferative process can assist in the exclusion of HCL. Lastly, although CD103 is the most specific of hairy cell antigens, the usefulness of this marker can be overstated because expression has been described in some cases of SMZL, which can mimic HCL clinically and cytologically.

The Royal Marsden group has developed several useful immunophenotypic scoring systems for differentiating B-cell lymphoproliferative disorders [21,22]. A four-point system for HCL uses CD103, CD11c, CD25, and another antibody with high specificity for HCL, HC2. Although HC2 is not used widely in the United States, a modified three-point system retains usefulness because SMZL and HCL-variant almost never coexpress CD103, CD11c, and CD25, whereas at least 90% of cases of HCL are positive for all three antigens [21].

Immunohistochemical studies
The wide accessibility to an ever-expanding library of antibodies and nearly universal use of trephine biopsy in bone marrow pathology have made immunohistochemical stains the primary ancillary tool in the diagnosis of HCL. Additionally, because a remarkable degree of marrow involvement by HCL can be inapparent in routinely stained histologic sections, immunohistochemical studies are requisite for adequate posttreatment evaluation for the efficacy of treatment.

Optimal immunohistochemical evaluation includes generic B-cell antibodies (CD20, CD79a, or PAX5) and markers with specificity for HCL, including TRAP, DBA.44, and cyclin D1. Generic B-cell markers, although lacking specificity for HCL, are highly sensitive and are useful for quantification of marrow involvement. CD20 is preferable because the thick granular membrane pattern is somewhat distinctive for HCL, and the lack of cytoplasmic or nuclear staining permits cytologic assessment of positive cells (Fig. 4A).

DBA.44, an antibody that originally was raised against a centroblastic cell line [23], was found incidentally to be a sensitive marker of HCL, and is expressed in 99% of cases [24]. The antibody displays a granular cytoplasmic pattern of expression and usually stains fewer cells than are demonstrated with

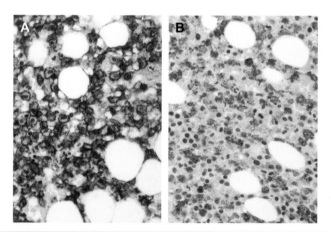

Fig. 4. (A) CD20 immunostain marks HCL with a characteristic thick and granular membrane pattern that permits cytologic assessment of the positive cells. Bone marrow (CD20 immunostain, original magnification ×40). (B) DBA.44 immunostain shows a granular cytoplasmic pattern of positivity and usually stains only a subset of the CD20 positive hairy cells. Bone marrow (CD20 immunostain, original magnification ×40).

CD20 (Fig. 4B). This antibody, although positive in less than 20% of other low grade B-cell lymphoproliferative diseases, unfortunately is expressed in up to 80% of cases of SMZL, which often is in the morphologic differential diagnosis of HCL [25]. DBA.44 also is expressed in a significant minority (20%–40%) of follicular lymphoma, mantle cell lymphoma (MCL), and diffuse large B-cell lymphoma [24].

Cytochemical staining for TRAP requires air-dried cytologic preparations and cannot be performed on paraffin-embedded tissue; however, antibodies that are specific for isoenzyme 5 of acid phosphatase have been developed in the last decade [26–28]. TRAP antibodies mark greater than 90% of cases of HCL and have sensitivity that is essentially equivalent to the cytochemical stain. Similar to DBA.44, this antibody has a granular cytoplasmic pattern and marks only a subset of the hairy cells, and, thus, is inferior to CD20 for quantification of marrow involvement. The immunohistochemical TRAP stain has a specificity that is significantly inferior to cytochemical TRAP and is reported to be positive in other lymphoproliferative disorders, including B-CLL/SLL, SMZL, and MCL [28,29]. As well, immunohistochemical TRAP is positive in several nonneoplastic cells, including osteoclasts, Gaucher cells, mast cells, and activated macrophages [27].

Cyclin D1 is overexpressed consistently in MCL, and has great usefulness in differentiating this intermediate-grade lymphoma from other low-grade mimics. Antibodies to this protein also mark nearly all cases of HCL with a dim nuclear pattern of staining in a subset of the hairy cells [30].

Immunohistochemical stains serve two primary purposes in the evaluation of HCL. First, a combination of DBA.44, TRAP, and cyclin D1 can be used to confirm a morphologic impression of HCL either in the setting of initial diagnosis or following chemotherapy in assessing a minor population of CD20-positive B cells. A DBA.44$^+$/TRAP$^+$ profile had a 97% specificity for HCL in a recent study [29]. Although not documented, it is likely that the addition of cyclin D1 to this panel would enhance specificity. Second, a CD20 immunostain is an excellent tool for quantification of an HCL infiltrate. This stain nearly always reveals more extensive disease than is evident from routinely stained sections and commonly shows persistent disease when hematoxylin-eosin–stained sections show no discernable infiltrate.

This discussion has focused on the use of immunohistochemical stains in bone marrow evaluation, because these specimens constitute most tissue biopsies that are performed on patients who have HCL. They are, of course, similarly useful in supporting a morphologic diagnosis of HCL in spleen, liver, lymph node, and other tissue samples.

TISSUE-SPECIFIC PATHOLOGY OF HAIRY CELL LEUKEMIA
Peripheral Blood
Abnormalities of the peripheral blood are identified at presentation in nearly all patients who have HCL. Pancytopenia is common, with neutropenia out of proportion to the degree of anemia and thrombocytopenia. Most distinctive

is a dearth of circulating monocytes, a finding so consistent that the diagnosis of HCL is unlikely in the absence of monocytopenia [31]. A note of caution in this regard: many automated hemogram analyzers categorize circulating hairy cells as monocytes. If present in sufficient number, they will mask monocytopenia unless a peripheral blood film is reviewed. The peripheral blood film often displays an increase in circulating large granular lymphocytes. These cells, with abundant gray-blue cytoplasm, can mimic the cytologic appearance of hairy cells. However, hairy cells rarely contain the sparse azurophilic granulation characteristic of large granular lymphocytes. Despite the near constant presence of reticulin myelofibrosis in HCL, leukoerythroblastosis usually is not prominent.

Circulating hairy cells are present in variable, usually low, numbers. In most cases a diligent search for cytologically typical hairy cells is required. This search should focus on the thin portions of the blood film. Although thicker portions of the smear accentuate the hairiness of the leukemic cells, this artifact-rich region commonly induces hairy projections of normal lymphocytes while obscuring most of the other characteristic cytologic features of HCL. When rare cells that are suggestive of HCL are identified in leukopenic peripheral blood films, buffy coat preparations often are useful in demonstrating additional hairy cells. As well, these concentrated smears greatly facilitate the interpretation of cytochemical acid phosphatase stains for evidence of TRAP positivity. Although the neoplastic cells in HCL are monotonous in appearance, most of them do not have classic "textbook" cytologic features. Hence, the reviewer commonly encounters several suspicious lymphocytes before encountering a cytologically classic hairy cell. Although leukopenia is the rule in HCL, a leukemic presentation, which is more characteristic of the variant form of HCL and SMZL, is encountered occasionally in patients who have otherwise typical HCL [32]. The peripheral blood film shows abnormal lymphocytosis with many classic hairy cells.

Bone Marrow

Infiltration of the bone marrow by HCL usually is accompanied by reticulin fibrosis, and the marrow often is deemed inaspirable [2]. The incidence of "dry tap" bone marrow aspiration likely is overstated, and reflects the common definition of "dry tap" as an inability to draw liquid bone marrow into the syringe; however, the bone marrow aspirate needle in "dry tap" aspirations often contains a few drops of blood that are rich in bone marrow elements. Expressing even minimal material from the needle directly onto glass slides often results in excellent cytologic preparations. A second alternative to standard bone marrow aspirate smears is the creation of touch preparations of the core biopsy, which should be prepared routinely with all bone marrow biopsies as a backup should the aspirate smears prove to be lacking in marrow particles [33]. If these two techniques are used, adequate cytologic preparations that permit identification of cytologically typical hairy cells and cytochemical staining for TRAP are available in most patients who have HCL. The mechanical stress of bone marrow aspiration or smear preparation, coupled with the fragility of the neoplastic cells in HCL, results in the presence of numerous nuclei that are stripped of cytoplasm and often outnumber intact hairy cells. In addition to infiltration with HCL, cytologic preparations of bone marrow specimens usually show erythroid-predominant hematopoiesis because of selective suppression of granulocytopoiesis [5].

Routinely stained histologic sections of bone marrow in HCL demonstrate a highly distinctive patchy or diffuse mononuclear infiltrate [3]. The aggregates are ill-defined and blend imperceptibly with surrounding residual hematopoiesis that usually is erythroid predominant. Unlike most other lymphoproliferative disorders, HCL demonstrates an infiltrative rather than "pushing" growth pattern that results in at least the focal preservation of marrow adipose tissue, despite extensive HCL surrounding fat lobules. Disruption of bone marrow microvasculature by hairy cell infiltrates results in the presence of extravasated erythrocytes. At low power, the infiltrates of HCL are paucicellular relative to other lymphoproliferative disorders, particularly B-CLL, SMZL, follicular lymphoma, and MCL. The well-spaced appearance is due to the abundant cytoplasm of hairy cells and to the pericellular deposition of fibronectin. Often, the infiltrates are paratrabecular and intramedullary in distribution and have an extremely monotonous appearance at medium power. The cells have round, oval, reniform, and lobated nuclei and the nuclear contours are not as smooth as in cytologic preparations. Chromatin is condensed partially and granular. The cells are without nucleoli or contain a single small nucleolus. Nuclei with features of transformed cells, including dispersed chromatin and prominent nucleoli, are virtually absent, as are mitotic figures. Cytoplasm is abundant and pale staining. The nuclei are placed centrally within the cytoplasmic domain, which imparts the well-spaced and monotonous appearance at medium power. The abundant and pale-staining cytoplasm surrounding smoothly contoured and round nuclei have inspired many observers to compare hairy cells with "fried eggs" (Fig. 5A). Infrequently, vague cytoplasmic condensations may be identified that represent large ribosome-lamella complexes.

When arrayed as sheets of monotonous cells, hairy cells are identified readily; however, in the context of surrounding hematopoietic elements, individual hairy cells in hematoxylin-eosin–stained sections closely mimic monocytes and myelocytes. Hence, when HCL infiltrates the marrow in an interstitial pattern it can be completely inapparent until immunostains highlight the subtle population of hairy cells.

The myelofibrosis that is associated with HCL represents deposition of fibronectin, which is synthesized and excreted by the hairy cells [34]. This likely explains the uniform pericellular increase in marrow reticulin that is demonstrated with silver stains. Occasional patients who have otherwise typical HCL have no evidence of reticulin deposition and easily aspirable bone marrow. Because the ground substance that is deposited in HCL is fibronectin, trichrome staining typically does not show deposition of mature collagen [35]. Occasional cases show prominent collagen deposition, however [36]. In these

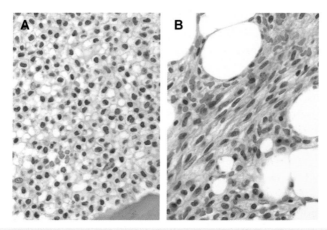

Fig. 5. (A) This is an image of the classic bone marrow infiltrate of HCL. The infiltrate is monotonous and the abundant cytoplasm imparts a well-spaced appearance to the centrally placed nuclei. Bone marrow (hematoxylin-eosin, original magnification ×40). (B) Marrow fibrosis can give a spindle-shaped appearance to the HCL infiltrate. Bone marrow (hematoxylin-eosin, original magnification ×40).

biopsies, fibroblasts are admixed with hairy cells that often take on a spindled fibroblastoid appearance (Fig. 5B). This morphologic variant of HCL must be differentiated from other fibrosing spindle cell proliferations in the bone marrow, and it can be mimicked closely by systemic mast cell disease (see "Differential diagnosis" below).

Occasionally, HCL simulates aplastic anemia [37] (Fig. 6). In this variant of the disease, patients present with pancytopenia and bone marrow biopsy demonstrates a markedly hypocellular medullary space. The infiltrate of hairy cells can be subtle and masked by admixed residual hematopoietic precursors. The

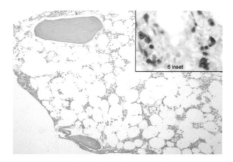

Fig. 6. HCL can present with pancytopenia and a markedly hypoplastic bone marrow that simulates aplastic anemia. Immunostain for CD20 (*inset*) shows a subtle infiltrate of hairy cells. Bone marrow (hematoxylin-eosin, original magnification ×4). Inset: Bone marrow (CD20 immunostain, original magnification ×40).

possibility of HCL should be considered in all adult patients who have apparent aplastic anemia. A CD20 immunostain is an easy and cost-effective way to evaluate for this neoplastic, but treatable, cause of marrow aplasia (Fig. 6, inset) [38].

There are several nonspecific changes associated with marrow infiltration by HCL. There often is an increase in polyclonal plasma cells [3]. Although a definite association between HCL and multiple myeloma has not been proven, multiple myeloma is a common disease among the elderly patient population that typically is afflicted with HCL, and occasional patients who have both diseases have been reported [39–41]. Hence, a significant degree of plasmacytosis, formation of plasma cell nodules, or atypical cytologic features should prompt immunostaining for evidence of immunoglobulin light-chain restriction to distinguish reactive plasmacytosis and multiple myeloma. An increase in marrow mast cells also is common in HCL [42]. The mast cells are mature, interstitial in distribution, and unlikely to suggest mast cell disease, although a single case of concomitant HCL and systemic mast cell disease has been reported [43]. Lastly, abnormal bone remodeling and lytic bone lesions have been described in rare cases of HCL [44].

Spleen

The pathology of the spleen in HCL is well described [2,45–47], reflecting the utility of therapeutic splenectomy before the development of effective chemotherapeutic strategies. However, splenectomy in HCL is now performed only infrequently.

HCL is a disease of the splenic red pulp that results in moderate to marked splenomegaly in nearly all patients. The expanded red pulp shows a variable degree of architectural effacement although sinuses and cords of Billroth—while infiltrated with hairy cells—usually are preserved. Hairy cell infiltrates generally are most prominent in the cords. The histologic appearance of the infiltrate is similar to that described in the bone marrow with a monotonous population of small- to intermediate-sized mononuclear cells with well-spaced nuclei and an absence of transformed cells and mitotic figures (Fig. 7A). Hairy cells infiltrate and replace sinus endothelium and result in degeneration of the sinus basement membrane, which requires endothelial support. Loss of the basement membrane results in dilation of the erythrocyte-filled vascular space, now lined by hairy cells, which creates the characteristic "blood lake" that typifies splenic involvement by HCL (Fig. 7B) [45]. In contrast to the marked red pulp expansion, the white pulp of the spleen frequently is hypoplastic. Although marrow fibrosis is common in HCL, splenic extramedullary hematopoiesis is encountered only infrequently and is not prominent.

Liver

Like the spleen, the hepatic pathology of HCL was well described in the era of therapeutic splenectomy when wedge biopsies of the liver were part of the standard surgical staging laparotomy for lymphoma [45,48,49]. Since that time,

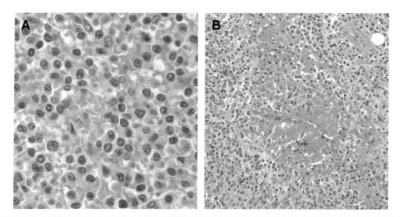

Fig. 7. (A) The spleen in HCL shows expansion of the red pulp with a monotonous population of cells that resembles the marrow infiltrates (hematoxylin-eosin, original magnification ×40). (B) The red pulp of the spleen is characterized by the formation of hairy cell–lined collections of erythrocytes that are referred to as "blood lakes" (hematoxylin-eosin, original magnification ×20).

liver biopsies involved by HCL have become a curiosity. Nevertheless, the liver is nearly always involved at presentation. Typically, hairy cells infiltrate the hepatic sinuses and portal tracts (Fig. 8, A and B). Sinus involvement often is subtle and is overlooked easily if HCL is not suspected. If a mononuclear infiltrate is recognized, immunostain for CD20 typically demonstrates that the hairy cell infiltrate is out of proportion to that suspected in routinely stained sections. When the portal tracts are involved, there is expansion of this compartment with a histologically characteristic infiltrate that permits ready recognition. A distinctive hepatic lesion in HCL is the "angiomatoid focus," which is composed of a congeries of apparent vascular spaces that mimic the appearance of a small vascular tumor but actually is composed of a collection of blood-filled spaces that are lined by hairy cells (Fig. 8C) [45]. The formation of these peculiar lesions is believed to be similar to the mechanism of blood lake formation in the spleen.

Lymph Node

Peripheral lymph node enlargement is rare in HCL; however, involvement of splenic hilar lymph nodes is common, and significant abdominal and retroperitoneal node involvement occurs in occasional patients. Such lymphadenopathy may be associated with atypical cytology and a more aggressive clinical course [50]. HCL infiltrates lymph node in a marginal zone or interfollicular pattern. Even when diffuse paracortical involvement is present, nodal sinuses often are preserved. The infiltrate has an appearance similar to that described in other organs. Although blood lake formation is rare, extravasated erythrocytes are common.

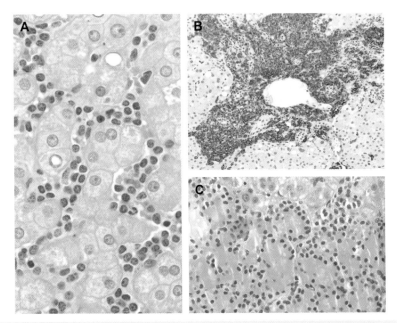

Fig. 8. (A) Liver involvement in HCL is characterized most commonly by sinus infiltration by the monotonous hairy cells (hematoxylin-eosin, original magnification ×40). (B) Occasionally the hepatic involvement is portal, as illustrated here with a CD20 immunostain that highlights the HCL infiltrate (original magnification ×10). (C) Rarely, an angiomatoid congeries of blood-filled spaces that are lined by hairy cells analogous to the splenic "blood lakes" is present. Liver (hematoxylin-eosin, original magnification ×20).

Other Tissues

Except for autopsy series that were reported before the advent of effective chemotherapy [51,52], involvement of tissues other than those discussed above is rare. Such oddities include reports of cutaneous involvement [53] and involvement of a hernia sac [54].

ASSESSMENT FOR RESIDUAL DISEASE

The pathologic assessment of patients who have HCL following 2-Chlorodeoxy adenosine (2-CdA) or other effective therapy has revealed that 15% to 50% of patients have demonstrable residual disease using moderately sensitive techniques, including immunohistochemistry and flow cytometry. Residual HCL that is detected by these methods and not evident with routine morphologic examination is termed minimal residual disease (MRD). Although the efficacy of minimal residual HCL for predicting clinical relapse has been suggested by several studies [55,56], it is evident that many patients who have MRD do not progress, or do so only over many years [57]. Hence, the predictive value of MRD detection in HCL is low and this finding has limited clinical usefulness at this time.

The limited usefulness of MRD detection does not obviate the need for ancillary techniques in the evaluation of follow-up bone marrows in patients who have HCL. The morphologic assessment of posttreatment bone marrow using routine histologic and cytologic stains is challenging. The interstitial pattern of disease and histologic resemblance of hairy cells to myelocytes and monocytes can mask residual HCL that composes as much as 10% of marrow cellularity. Hence, immunostains are a critical component of the posttherapy evaluation of HCL to ferret out and reproducibly quantify residual disease. Although many studies have defined relapse or persistent disease as the identification of HCL in routine stains [55,57], the ability to recognize residual HCL is dependent on the experience of the reviewing pathologist. This standard may be suitable in institutions that care for a large number of patients who have HCL, but it is unrealistic for those that rarely encounter HCL. Much as CD138 immunostains have become the method of choice for quantification of multiple myeloma, CD20 or DBA.44 staining serves as an accessible and reproducible method for identifying and quantifying hairy cells; the routine use of these immunostains, although not essential, is justifiable. If immunohistochemical or flow cytometry studies are not performed, the pathologic interpretation should specify that a small amount of residual disease cannot be excluded.

An important caveat in the routine use of these immunostains is the recognition that a small number of CD20- and DBA.44-positive cells, some resembling hairy cells, are present in normal bone marrow [58]. Hence, the findings generally should be considered nondiagnostic when the population of immunohistochemically identified mononuclear cells composes less than 5% of marrow cellularity, and there is no additional supportive evidence of residual disease, such as cytochemical TRAP-positive cells or flow cytometric evidence of monoclonal B cells with a characteristic phenotype. Because the literature lacks clarity regarding morphologic criteria for relapse and the clinical significance of a minor population of clinically inapparent HCL, a cautious approach is to deem 5% to 10% populations as suspicious for HCL and to reserve definitive diagnosis of HCL for when cytologically appropriate B cells exceed 10% of marrow cellularity.

THE DIFFERENTIAL DIAGNOSIS OF HAIRY CELL LEUKEMIA

The initial diagnostic specimens in patients who have HCL rarely are submitted to the pathology department with a clinical history of "Rule out hairy cell leukemia." Hence, it is important to discuss the broad range of diagnoses that must be considered and excluded in the evaluation of this often clinically obscure disease.

Cytopathologic Differential Diagnosis

The classic cytologic appearance of the hairy cell is distinctive and the presence of numerous characteristic cells is diagnostic of HCL independent of any supportive studies. Unfortunately, HCL often presents with a dearth of evaluable cells, suboptimal cytologic preparations, or a predominance of cells lacking diagnostic features. These settings raise alternative diagnostic considerations.

HCL-V, discussed below, is characterized by cells that can resemble typical HCL (Fig. 9). Shared features include cell size, nuclear contours, and a moderate to abundant rim of cytoplasm with cytoplasmic projections. In contrast to HCL, the cells of HCL-V typically have a single prominent nucleolus, more chromatin condensation, and cells with basophilic cytoplasm. As well, the neoplastic cells of HCL-V tend to be polymorphous relative to the consistent monotony of HCL.

SMZL, also known as splenic lymphoma with villous lymphocytes can resemble HCL; they share an abundant rim of cytoplasm and cytoplasmic projections (Fig. 10A). The nuclear chromatin in SMZL usually is more condensed and irregularly distributed than in HCL. The cytoplasm lacks the characteristic flocculent appearance of the classic hairy cell and often is more basophilic. Villous lymphocytes typically have well-defined cytoplasmic margins without the frayed appearance that is seen in HCL. Lastly, when projections are present, they tend to be polar and blunt, in contrast to the thin and circumferential "hairs" that typify HCL.

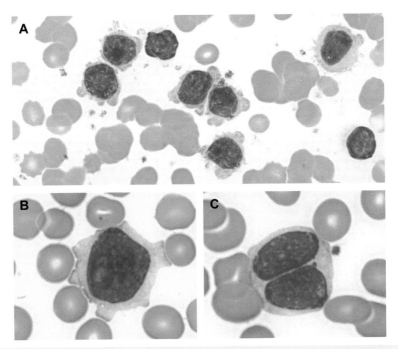

Fig. 9. (A) HCL-V commonly presents with leukocytosis in contrast to the dearth of hairy cells that typifies the peripheral blood of typical HCL. Peripheral blood (Wright's stain, original magnification ×100). (B) This is a characteristic cell of HCL-V. Note the prominent nucleolus, smudgy chromatin, and lack of the textured, flocculent cytoplasm of typical HCL. Peripheral blood (Wright's stain, original magnification ×100). (C) Unusual nuclear configurations, such as this binucleate form, often are present in HCL-V. Peripheral blood (Wright's stain, original magnification ×100).

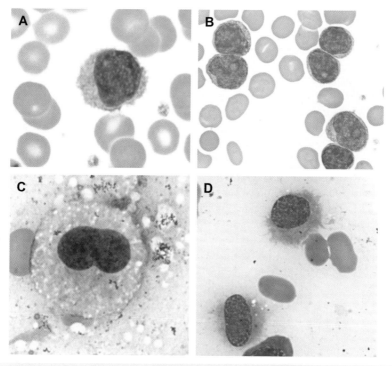

Fig. 10. (A) SMZL can have cells that mimic typical HCL; however, the cells in this disease have smudgy chromatin, more cytoplasmic basophilia, and blunt polar cytoplasmic projections. Peripheral blood (Wright's stain, original magnification ×100). (B) Prolymphocytic leukemia has an appearance that more closely resembles HCL-V than typical HCL. Peripheral blood (Wright's stain, original magnification ×100). (C) Rare cases of multiple myeloma have, in addition to typical myeloma cells (not illustrated), a population of cells that closely resembles HCL. Bone marrow (Wright's stain, original magnification ×100). (D) Agranular mast cells in systemic mast cell disease have nuclear characteristics that closely mimic HCL; however, the cytoplasm has a tan-blue color and the cells lack cytoplasmic projections. Bone marrow (Wright's stain, original magnification ×100).

Cells with an unusually generous rim of cytoplasm that bear some resemblance to HCL can characterize B-CLL and B-cell prolymphocytic leukemia (Fig. 10B). Nuclear features, especially the distinctive "ginger snap" chromatin pattern of B-CLL and the presence of a minor population of prolymphocytes, usually permit ready distinction from HCL.

From the relatively informed perspective of the twenty-first century, it is important to recognize that the hairy cell has cytologic features that are more akin to a monocyte than to a mature lymphocyte. The descriptive nature of the moniker "hairy cell leukemia" supplanted the earlier term "leukemic reticuloendotheliosis" specifically to reflect the ambiguous lineage of the neoplastic cells that remained unresolved until the 1980s [5,59]. Acute monocytic leukemia (AML-M5b in the French-American-British [FAB] system) occasionally shows differentiation toward a distinctive cell type that is referred to as a plasmacytoid monocyte. These cells have round or oval nuclei without the characteristic folding of typical monocytes. The abundant rim of cytoplasm generally is agranular and lacks vacuolization. Moreover, the cells are fragile with numerous ruptured cells in cytologic preparations. Hence, these cells can resemble HCL reflected in the conflation of monocytic leukemia and HCL in early publications [2,60]. The immature chromatin of these atypical promonocytes and occasional forms with sparse azurophilic granulation assist in the cytologic discrimination from hairy cells.

The neoplastic cells in systemic mast cell disease can be devoid of the metachromatic granules that crowd the cytoplasm of normal mast cells. These agranular forms display nuclear features that are remarkably similar to HCL with round, oval, reniform, and dumbbell-shaped nuclei and partially condensed, evenly dispersed chromatin (Fig. 10C). The abundant cytoplasm also is similar to hairy cells; however, mast cells have well-defined cytoplasmic borders and lack hairy projections. As well, careful review usually reveals the presence of some cells with at least sparse granulation.

Finally, rare cases of multiple myeloma display a subset of neoplastic cells that is virtually indistinguishable from HCL (Fig. 10D) [61]. Although the clinical context and admixed typical myeloma cells seem to permit ready distinction from true hairy cells, the two diseases occasionally occur synchronously, an intriguing, but likely coincidental association. Careful review for cells with intermediate features of myeloma and HCL favors an interpretation of multiple myeloma with hairy cell–like features, but flow cytometry may be required to evaluate for concomitant HCL.

Histopathologic Differential Diagnosis

The diffuse monotonous infiltrate of small- to intermediate-sized mononuclear cells with well-spaced nuclei that is characteristic of HCL is mimicked by several other malignant infiltrates. Marginal zone lymphoma (splenic, extranodal, or nodal) with monocytoid B cells can be indistinguishable from HCL in routinely stained sections. HCL-V has a similar low- and medium-power appearance to typical HCL, although the cytologic features of this disease usually permit distinction. Mast cell disease can bear a close resemblance to HCL, although mast cell infiltrates tend to be more discrete than HCL. Admixed eosinophils are an important clue to the diagnosis of systemic mast cell disease. Two forms of acute myeloid leukemia, acute monocytic leukemia (AML-M5b) and acute promyelocytic leukemia (AML-M3), are characterized by monotonous sheets of cells with a well-spaced appearance. Like HCL, the nuclear contours frequently are reniform to bilobed; however, the immature chromatin pattern and numerous mitotic figures of these disorders usually permit ready distinction from HCL. Lastly, several types of metastatic disease enter the "monotonous well-spaced nuclei" differential diagnosis, particularly lobular carcinoma of the breast and malignant melanoma.

Tissue-Specific Considerations

Bone marrow

In the evaluation of bone marrow infiltrates, there are several features that assist in the morphologic differential diagnosis. Although SMZL can have a monocytoid appearance that mimics HCL, there often is a small lymphocytic component with lymphoid aggregates of tightly packed small lymphocytes similar to those of B-CLL that are not a feature of HCL. As well, SMZL often displays a sinusoidal growth pattern and the occasional presence of benign germinal centers, two features that help in distinction from HCL. Mast cell infiltrates tend to be circumscribed relative to the ill-defined hairy cell aggregates, often are paratrabecular, and have associated eosinophils.

Spleen

The exclusive red pulp pattern of splenic HCL is a useful feature in differential diagnosis. SMZL, MCL, and follicular lymphoma principally involve the white pulp; red pulp involvement, if present, usually has a micronodular appearance that reflects expansion of the periarteriolar lymphoid sheaths. Hence, these disorders are distinguished readily from HCL. Mast cell disease involves the spleen in a patchy manner with most aggregates at the red/white pulp interface; it is not a significant consideration, despite the similarities discussed above. B-CLL typically involves red and white pulp, which results in blurring of the margins between these two compartments. Although this pattern of involvement can resemble HCL, the expanded white pulp and tightly packed small lymphocytic infiltrate of B-CLL/SLL usually permits ready distinction.

Lymphoproliferative disorders that are characterized by a pure red pulp pattern include HCL, HCL-V, hepatosplenic T-cell lymphoma, and rare cases of SMZL. HCL-V can mimic the classic histologic pattern of HCL, including diffuse red pulp involvement with the formation of blood lakes that are lined by neoplastic cells. Recognition of the atypical cytologic features is the only morphologic means of distinguishing these disorders. SMZL with a red pulp pattern [62] lacks blood lake formation and usually contain a variable number of transformed cells that are absent in HCL. Parenthetically, the distinction between HCL-V and the red pulp variant of SMZL is a greater challenge than is distinguishing either of these disorders from HCL; it requires characterization of the neoplastic cells with flow cytometry. Hepatosplenic T-cell lymphoma is an aggressive process with an atypical histologic appearance and high proliferative rate that does not mimic the cytologic appearance of HCL. Lastly, acute leukemia is characterized by involvement of the splenic red pulp. Hence, acute monocytic leukemia (AML-M5b) can mimic HCL in the spleen; however, monocytic leukemia lacks the blood lakes of HCL and usually has immature nuclear features and mitotic figures.

Resolution of Morphologic Differential Diagnoses

The above discussion of differential diagnosis is directed toward the initial morphologic evaluation of tissue samples from patients who do not have a pre-existing diagnosis of HCL. Resolution of these considerations is based on the application of a panel of cytochemistry, flow cytometry, or immunohisto-chemistry studies to demonstrate the diagnostic characteristics of HCL that were described in detail above. Additionally, a focused battery of tests to exclude other diagnostic possibilities should be performed, although the specifics of this evaluation vary depending on the specific pathologic findings and are beyond the scope of this discussion.

CATEGORIZATION OF HAIRY CELL LEUKEMIA AND RELATED DISORDERS

The following categorization is suggested in the evaluation of low-grade B-cell lymphoproliferative disorders with features that are characteristic of, or closely related to, HCL:

HCL
  Typical
  With unusual features:
    Clinical
    Cytologic
    Immunophenotypic
  HCL-V
  SMZL
  Low-grade B-cell lymphoproliferative disorder, HCL-V versus SMZL

Hairy Cell Leukemia

"Typical HCL" is applied to lymphoproliferative disorders with cytologic and histologic features that are characteristic of HCL. It is first and foremost, a morphologic diagnosis. Some degree of ancillary testing is desirable to confirm a morphologic diagnosis and may include cytochemical staining for TRAP, immunophenotypic analysis by flow cytometry, and immunohistochemical stains. In a morphologically typical case, only one or two of these modalities is necessary to confirm a diagnosis of HCL.

As illustrated in the list above, the subcategory of "HCL with unusual features" is used to highlight cases of HCL that have some atypical characteristic. The presence of an unusual feature should prompt a more extensive panel of ancillary studies than for typical HCL. This panel must generate findings that are consonant with a diagnosis of HCL. Atypical clinical characteristics include isolated skeletal lesions [63,64], leukemia cutis [65], retroperitoneal mass [50], or significant leukocytosis [32]. Cytologically unusual cases generally include otherwise typical hairy cells of large size [9] or cells that demonstrate exaggerated nuclear configurations, including numerous horseshoe-shaped, spindled, or lobated forms [7,8]. Immunophenotypically unusual cases show some phenotypic characteristics that stray from the expected, including expression of CD10 or lack of one of the signature hairy cell markers (bright CD11c, CD25, CD103). Despite these clinical, cytologic, or immunophenotypic deviations, these cases can be categorized unequivocally as "HCL." The atypical features can be elaborated in the interpretive comment.

Variant Form of Hairy Cell Leukemia

In stark contrast to the clearly defined criteria and unique characteristics of HCL, HCL-V lacks such well-limned contours. This rare disease, at least 10-fold less common than HCL [66,67], has features that suggest to varying degrees HCL, SMZL, and prolymphocytic leukemia. The perplexity of this borderline lesion is heightened by the relationship to the similarly ill-defined prolymphocytic leukemia and an irresolvable overlap in some patients who have SMZL. As well, from a terminology perspective, "HCL-V" invites confusion with cases of HCL with atypical features as described above. This distinction is not trivial because patients who have HCL-V have significantly inferior response to 2-CdA and other effective HCL treatment strategies [66–68]. Add to this the existence of a Japanese variant form of HCL and there is a "perfect storm" of confusion that swirls around HCL-V. In such a morass, it is useful to ask, "Is there a set of clinical and pathologic criteria that permits diagnostic certitude on par with that of other lymphoproliferative disorders?". This discussion attempts to demonstrate an affirmative answer to that query and briefly explores the approach to borderline lesions.

Clinical characteristics of the variant form of hairy cell leukemia

HCL-V presents at an older age than does HCL (eighth versus sixth decades), and shows only a modest male predominance (<2:1) that contrasts with the 5:1 male/female distribution of HCL. Patients present with splenomegaly, lymphocytosis, and cytopenias, particularly anemia and thrombocytopenia. In contrast to HCL, monocytopenia and neutropenia are not features of HCL-V. Hence, the clinical presentation of HCL-V is unlike HCL and resembles SMZL [68].

Pathologic characteristics of the variant form of hairy cell leukemia

Cytopathology. The neoplastic cells of HCL-V are intermediate in size with nuclei that generally are round and have partially condensed chromatin that lacks the regular distribution of HCL and tends to have a smudged appearance (see Fig. 9). The cells often have a single medium to large nucleolus, although it recently was suggested that this cytologic feature may have been overemphasized and is not always present [69]. The cytoplasm is abundant with an appearance that is more basophilic and uniform than that of HCL with cytoplasmic margins that are well defined. Some cells have villous or hairlike projections. The cells lack the monotony of HCL and there are cell-to-cell variations in cytoplasmic basophilia, chromatin condensation, and nucleoli. As well, occasional transformed-appearing large cells may be present [68].

Ancillary studies. TRAP staining in HCL-V is variable and may be negative, brightly positive as in HCL, or show uniform dim positivity. Flow cytometry generally shows monoclonal B-cells that lack expression of CD5 and CD10. The cells predictably express CD11c, whereas about 60% express CD103. HCL-V is almost always negative for CD25. Immunohistochemical studies typically show expression of generic B-cell antigens. DBA.44 usually is positive [68,69]. A rare report [70] and a single evaluated case at Scripps Clinic (personal observation) indicate that the cells can express cyclin D1 in a manner similar to typical HCL.

Histopathology. The histopathology of HCL-V essentially mimics that of HCL, except for the differing cytologic characteristics. Specifically, the marrow infiltrates have the ill-defined and well-spaced appearance that typifies HCL, although fibrosis generally is mild or absent. There may be a sinusoidal growth pattern of infiltration [69]. As well, the selective granulocytic hypoplasia that characterizes HCL is not typical of HCL-V. In the spleen, HCL-V shows a red pulp pattern and some cases have "blood lake" formation. Hepatic involvement in HCL-V is likewise similar to HCL with sinusoidal and portal tract involvement [68].

Natural history
HCL-V tends to follow a more aggressive clinical course than does HCL and generally is less responsive to chemotherapy. The median survival is about a decade from diagnosis. As well, and in contrast to typical HCL, about 5% to 10% of cases of HCL-V undergo morphologic transformation to a large cell process that otherwise retains immunophenotypic characteristics of HCL-V. This transformation is associated with marked leukocytosis, B symptoms, and short survival [66,68].

Categorization of Cases in the Variant Form of Hairy Cell Leukemia/Splenic Marginal Zone Lymphoma Spectrum

A survey of the literature of HCL-V makes evident that there is no uniformity of diagnostic criteria, particularly in the distinction between HCL-V and SMZL. In this murky context, a conservative approach to the diagnosis of HCL-V is recommended. Definitive categorization of a lymphoproliferative process as HCL-V is warranted when a population of cytologically characteristic cells is present, including the uniform presence of prominent nucleoli. The lymphocytes must display an appropriate immunophenotypic profile characterized by expression of CD11c and a lack CD25. If the cytologic features are ambiguous with an admixture of cells that suggest both HCL-V and SMZL, a diagnosis of HCL-V should be reserved for patients with a characteristic phenotypic profile as well as bone marrow and splenic findings (including a red pulp pattern of splenic involvement) that resemble typical HCL. Alternatively, when only bone marrow biopsy is available, immunohistochemical evidence of cyclin D1 overexpression can be used to distinguish HCL-V from SMZL, as the latter should always be cyclin D1 negative. In the setting of a lymphoproliferative disorder that meets neither the above criteria nor those for SMZL, it is prudent to classify the process as "low-grade B-cell lymphoproliferative disorder, SMZL, or HCL-V."

SUMMARY

The pathology of HCL has been reviewed with a focus on the diagnostic hematopathology of this rare, but fascinating, disease. The discrimination of HCL from other B-cell lymphoproliferations, particularly HCL-V and SMZL, has been emphasized. The unique responsiveness of HCL to 2-CdA and other chemotherapeutic agents makes this distinction critical. Fortunately, HCL has consistent cytologic, histologic, cytochemical, and immunologic features that make classification reliable and reproducible. Less straightforward is the differential diagnosis of SMZL and HCL-V, problematic because of the rarity of both disorders, lack of discriminating evidence-based criteria, and perhaps a biologic kinship between these two disorders that share many clinical and pathologic features. Fortunately, this is not a clinically critical distinction.

References

[1] Yam LT, Li CY, Finkel HE. Leukemic reticuloendotheliosis. The role of tartrate-resistant acid phosphatase in diagnosis and splenectomy in treatment. Arch Int Med 1972;130:248–60.
[2] Bouroncle BA, Wiseman BK, Doan CA. Leukemia reticuloendothesliosis. Blood 1958; 13(7):609–30.
[3] Catovsky D, Pettit JE, Galton DAG, et al. Leukaemic reticuloendotheliosis ('hairy cell leukaemia'): a distinct clinico-pathologic entity. Br J Haematol 1974;26:9–27.
[4] Mitus WJ, Mednicoff IB, Wittels B, et al. Neoplastic lymphoid reticulum cells in the peripheral blood: a histochemical study. Blood 1961;17:206–14.
[5] Schrek R, Donnelly WJ. "Hairy" cells in the blood in lymphoreticular neoplastic disease and "flagellated" cells of normal lymph nodes. Blood 1966;27(2):199–211.
[6] Katayam I, Nagy GK, Balogh K. Light microscopic identification of the ribosome-lamella compex in "hairy cells" of leukemic reticuloendotheliosis. Cancer 1973;32:843–6.
[7] Invernizzi R, Castello A. A hairy cell leukemia variant with unusual nuclear morphology. Haematologica 1994;79:567–8.
[8] Hanson CA, Ward PCJ, Schnitzer B. A multilobular variant of hairy cell leukemia with morphologic similarities to T-cell lymphoma. Am J Surg Pathol 1989;13(8):671–9.
[9] Sun X, Amin HM, Freireich EJ, et al. Hairy cell leukemia with large cells: long disease course with adequate response to therapy. Leukemia 2004;18:1912–4.
[10] Katayama I, Li CY, Yam LT. Ultrastructural characteristics of "hairy cells" of leukemic reticuloendotheliosis. Am J Pathol 1972;67:361–70.
[11] Schnitzer B, Kass L. Hairy-cell leukemia. Am J Clin Pathol 1974;61:176–87.
[12] Katayama I, Schneider GB. Further ultrastructural characterization of hairy cells of leukemic reticuloendotheliosis. Am J Pathol 1977;86:163–82.
[13] Burke JS, Mackay B, Rappaport H. Hairy cell leukemia (leukemic reticuloendotheliosis) II. Ultrastructure of the spleen. Cancer 1976;37:2267–74.
[14] Yam LT, Li CY, Lam KW. Tartrate-resistant acid phosphatase isoenzyme in the reticulum cells of leukemic reticuloendotheliosis. N Engl J Med 1971;284:357–60.
[15] Usui T, Konishi H, Sawada H, et al. Existence of tartrate-resistant acid phosphatase activity in differentiated lymphoid leukemic cells. Am J Hematol 1982;12:47–54.
[16] Neiman RS, Sullivan AL, Jaffe R. Malignant lymphoma simulating leukemic reticuloendotheliosis. Cancer 1979;43:329–42.
[17] Sausville JE, Salloum RG, Sorbara L, et al. Minimal residual disease detection in hairy cell leukemia. Am J Clin Pathol 2003;119:213–7.
[18] von Bockstaele DR, Berneman ZN, Peetermans ME. Flow cytometric analysis of hairy cell leukemia using right-angle light scatter. Cytometry 1986;7:217–20.
[19] Jasionowski TM, Hartung L, Greenwood JH, et al. Analysis of CD10+ hairy cell leukemia. Am J Clin Pathol 2003;120:228–35.
[20] Robbins BA, Ellison DJ, Spinosa JC, et al. Diagnostic application of two-color flow cytometry in 161 cases of hairy cell leukemia. Blood 1993;82:1277–87.

[21] Matutes E, Morilla R, Owusu-Ankomah K, et al. The immunophenotype of hairy cell leukemia (HCL). Proposal for a scoring system to distinguish HCL from B-cell disorders with hairy or villous lymphocytes. Leuk Lymphoma 1994;14(Suppl 1):57–61.

[22] Matutes E, Owusu-Ankomah K, Morilla R, et al. The immunological profile of B-cell disorders and proposal of a scoring system for the diagnosis of CLL. Leukemia 1994;8:1640–5.

[23] Al Saati T, Caspar S, Brousset P, et al. Production of anti-B monoclonal antibodies (DBB.42, DBA.44, DNA.7, and DND.53) reactive on paraffin-embedded tissues with a new B-lymphoma cell line grafted into athymic nude mice. Blood 1989;74:2476–85.

[24] Hounieu H, Chittal SM, Al Saati T, et al. Hairy cell leukemia: diagnosis of bone marrow involvement in paraffin-embedded sections with monoclonal antibody DBA.44. Am J Clin Pathol 1992;98:26–33.

[25] Salomon-Nguyen F, Valensi F, Troussard X, et al. The value of the monoclonal antibody DBA.44 in the diagnosis of B-lymphoid disorders. Leuk Res 1996;20:909–13.

[26] Janckila AJ, Cardwell EM, Yam LT, et al. Hairy cell identification by immunohistochemistry of tartrate-resistant acid phosphatase. Blood 1995;85:2939–44.

[27] Yaziji H, Janckila AJ, Lear SC, et al. Immunohistochemical detection of tartrate-resistant acid phosphatase in non-hematopoietic human tissues. Am J Clin Pathol 1995;104:397–402.

[28] Hoyer JD, Li CY, Yam YT, et al. Immunohistochemical demonstration of acid phosphatase isoenzyme 5 (tartrate-resistant) in paraffin sections of hairy cell leukemia and other hematologic disorders. Am J Clin Pathol 1997;108:308–15.

[29] Went PT, Zimpfer A, Pehrs AC, et al. High specificity of combined TRAP and DBA.44 expression for hairy cell leukemia. Am J Surg Pathol 2005;29:474–8.

[30] Miranda RN, Briggs RC, Kinney MC, et al. Immunohistochemical detection of cyclin D1 using optimized conditions is highly specific for mantle cell lymphoma and hairy cell leukemia. Mod Pathol 2000;13:1308–14.

[31] Seshardri RS, Brown EJ, Zipursky A. Leukemic reticuloendotheliosis: a failure of monocyte production. N Engl J Med 1976;295:181–4.

[32] Adley BP, Sun X, Shaw JM, et al. Hairy cell leukemia with marked lymphocytosis. Arch Pathol Lab Med 2003;127:253–4.

[33] Krause JR, Srodes C, Lee RE. Use of the bone marrow imprint in the diagnosis of leukemic reticuloendotheliosis ("hairy cell leukemia"). Am J Clin Pathol 1977;68:368–71.

[34] Burthem J, Cawley JC. The bone marrow fibrosis of hairy-cell leukemia is caused by the synthesis of a fibronectin matrix by the hairy cells. Blood 1994;83:497–504.

[35] Naeim F, Smith GS. Leukemic reticuloendotheliosis. Cancer 1974;34:1813–21.

[36] Anderson RE, Walford RL. Fibroblastic type of leukemic reticuloendotheliosis. Cancer 1963;16:993–7.

[37] Lee WM, Beckstead JH. Hairy cell leukemia with bone marrow hypoplasia. Cancer 1982;50:2207–10.

[38] Ng JP, Nolan B, Chan-Lam D, et al. Successful treatment of aplastic variant of hairy-cell leukaemia with deoxycoformycin. Hematology (Am Soc Hematol Educ Program) 2002;7:259–62.

[39] Saif MW, Greenberg BR. Multiple myeloma and hairy cell leukemia: a rare association or coincidence? Leuk Lymphoma 2001;42:1043–8.

[40] Aronowitz J, Baral E, Dalal BI. Late transition of hairy cell leukemia to multiple myeloma. Am J Hematol 1993;44:216.

[41] Catovsky D, Costello C, Loukopoulos D, et al. Hairy cell leukemia and myelomatosis: chance association or clinical manifestations of the same B-cell disease spectrum. Blood 1981;57:758–63.

[42] Macon WR, Kinney MC, Glick AD, et al. Marrow mast cell hyperplasia in hairy cell leukemia. Mod Pathol 1993;6:695–8.

[43] Petrella T, Depret O, Arnould L, et al. Systemic mast cell disease associated with hairy cell leukaemia. Leuk Lymphoma 1997;25:593–5.

[44] Marcelli C, Chappard D, Rossi JF, et al. Histologic evidence of an abnormal bone remodeling in B cell malignancies other than multiple myeloma. Cancer 1988;62:1163–70.

[45] Nanba K, Soban EJ, Bowling MC, et al. Splenic pseudosinuses and hepatic angiomatous lesions. Distinctive features of hairy cell leukemia. Am J Clin Pathol 1977;67:415–26.

[46] Nanba K, Jaffe ES, Soban EJ, et al. Hairy cell leukemia. Enzyme histochemical characterization, with special reference to splenic stromal changes. Cancer 1977;39:2323–36.

[47] Pilon VA, Davey FR, Gordon GB. Splenic alterations in hairy cell leukemia. Arch Pathol Lab Med 1981;105:577–81.

[48] Roquet JL, Zafrani ES, Farcet JP, et al. Histopathological lesions of the liver in hairy cell leukemia; a report of 14 cases. Hepatology 1985;5:496–500.

[49] Yam LT, Janckila AJ, Chan CH, et al. Hepatic involvement in hairy cell leukemia. Cancer 1983;51:1497–504.

[50] Mercieca J, Matutes E, Moskovic E, et al. Massive abdominal lymphadenopathy in hairy cell leukemia: a report of 12 cases. Br J Haematol 1992;82:547–54.

[51] Vardiman JW, Golomb HM. Autopsy findings in hairy cell leukemia. Sem Oncol 1984;11:370–80.

[52] Vardiman JW, Variakojis D, Golomb HM. Hairy cell leukemia: an autopsy study. Cancer 1979;43:1339–49.

[53] Arai E, Ikeda S, Itoh S, et al. Specific skin lesions as the presenting symptom of hairy cell leukemia. Am J Clin Pathol 1988;90:459–64.

[54] Melaragno MJ, Theil KS, Marsh WL, et al. Hairy cell leukemia involving an inguinal hernial sac. Acta Haematol 1990;84:204–6.

[55] Wheaton S, Tallman MS, Hakimian D, et al. Minimal residual disease may predict bone marrow relapse in patients with hairy cell leukemia treated with 2-chlorodeoxyadenosine. Blood 1996;87:1556–60.

[56] Matutes E, Meeus K, McLennen K, et al. The significance of minimal residual disease in hairy cell leukemia treated with deoxycoformycin: a long-term follow-up study. Br J Haematol 1997;98:375–83.

[57] Ellison DJ, Sharpe RW, Robbins BA, et al. Immunomorphologic analysis of bone marrow biopsies after treatment with 2-chlorodeoxyadenosine for hairy cell leukemia. Blood 1994;84:4310–5.

[58] O'Donnell LR, Alder SL, Balis UJ, et al. Immunohistochemical reference ranges for B lymphocytes in bone marrow biopsy paraffin sections. Am J Clin Pathol 1995;104:517–23.

[59] Plenderleith IH. Hairy cell leukemia. J Can Med Assoc 1970;102:1056–60.

[60] Vaithianathan T, Bolonik SJ, Gruhn JG. Leukemic reticuloendotheliosis. Am J Clin Pathol 1962;38:605–14.

[61] Algino KM, Hendrix LE, Henderson CA, et al. Multiple myeloma with hairy cell-like features. Am J Clin Pathol 1997;107:665–71.

[62] Mollejo M, Algara P, Mateo MS, et al. Splenic small B-cell lymphoma with predominant red pulp involvement: a diffuse variant of splenic marginal zone lymphoma? Histopathol 2002;40:22–30.

[63] Demanes DJ, Lane N, Beckstead JH. Bone involvement in hairy-cell leukemia. Cancer 1982;49:1697–701.

[64] Lal A, Tallman MS, Soble MB, et al. Hairy cell leukemia presenting as localized skeletal involvement. Leuk Lymphoma 2002;43:2207–11.

[65] Bilsland D, Shahriari S, Douglas WS, et al. Transient leukaemia cutis in hairy-cell leukemia. Clin Exp Dermatol 1991;16:207–9.

[66] Matutes E, Wotherspoon A, Brito-Babapulle V, et al. The natural history and clinicopathological features of the variant form of hairy cell leukemia. Leukemia 2001;15:184–6.

[67] Tetreault SA, Robbins BA, Saven A. Treatment of hairy cell leukemia-variant with cladribine. Leuk Lymphoma 1999;35:347–54.

[68] Matutes E, Wotherspoon A, Catovsky D. The variant form of hairy cell leukemia. Best Pract Res Clin Haematol 2003;16:41–56.

[69] Cessna MH, Hartung L, Tripp S, et al. Hairy cell leukemia variant: fact or fiction. Am J Clin Pathol 2005;123:132–8.

[70] Bosch F, Campo E, Jares P, et al. Increased expression of the PRAD-1/CCND1 gene in hairy cell leukaemia. Br J Haematol 1995;91:1025–30.

HEMATOLOGY/ONCOLOGY CLINICS
OF NORTH AMERICA

SEVIER
UNDERS

Immunophenotyping and Differential Diagnosis of Hairy Cell Leukemia

Estella Matutes, MD, PhD

Department of Haemato-Oncology, The Royal Marsden Hospital and Institute of Cancer Research, 203 Fulham Road, London, SW3 6JJ, UK

Hairy cell leukemia (HCL) is an uncommon mature B-cell lymphoproliferative disorder that was described first in the late 1950s [1]. The disease has distinct clinical features, morphology, histopathology, and immunophenotype [2]. Although the monocytic versus lymphoid cell origin in HCL had been debated for several years, immunologic markers were instrumental in establishing the lymphoid origin of the hairy cells by the demonstration of the expression of immunoglobulin (Ig) heavy and light chains in their cell surface. The lymphoid nature was confirmed and substantiated by molecular analysis that showed rearrangement of the Ig heavy-chain genes in the neoplastic cells [3].

A variant form of HCL (HCL-variant) in which the cells appear to have an intermediate morphology between a hairy cell and a prolymphocyte was documented first in 1982 [4]. This disease was described later in small series of patients [5,6], and has been recognized by the World Health Organization [2]. HCL-variant has splenic and bone marrow pathologic features that are similar or identical to typical HCL; however, the clinical course, response to treatment, cell morphology, and immunophenotype is different from that seen in the typical HCL. Because of the different outcomes of typical HCL and HCL-variant, a distinction between the two diseases becomes a relevant clinical issue.

This article describes the immunophenotypic characteristics of the tissue (bone marrow and spleen) infiltrating and circulating blood cells from patients who have typical HCL and HCL-variant, and discusses the differential diagnosis of these disorders with other lymphoid and nonlymphoid conditions.

DIAGNOSTIC IMMUNOPHENOTYPING
Hairy Cell Leukemia

Before the advent of the monoclonal antibodies (McAb's), a useful and widely used test for the diagnosis of HCL was standard cytochemistry that investigated the reactivity for the acid phosphatase enzyme, which in the case of hairy cells, is resistant to tartaric acid (TRAP$^+$). This hydrolase corresponds to the

E-mail address: estella.matutes@icr.ac.uk

0889-8588/06/$ – see front matter
doi:10.1016/j.hoc.2006.06.012

isoenzyme 5 of the acid phosphatase [7]. Although TRAP is not exclusive to hairy cells because it is present in cells from the mononuclear phagocytic system as well as in mitogen-activated normal B cells, in the context of lymphoid neoplasms, particularly those derived from B cells, it seems to be almost unique to HCL [8]. A McAb against TRAP is available and its use by immunohistochemistry on tissue sections in combination with DBA44 has proved to be useful for diagnostic purposes [9].

The phenotype of the hairy cell appears to be that of an activated memory B cell with aberrant expression of genes that control cell adhesion and response to cytokines [10]. The postgerminal center origin of the hairy cell also was suggested by studies that investigated the mutational status of the Ig heavy-chain genes and by microarray gene expression [10,11]. Furthermore, and reinforcing this hypothesis, antigens that are lost following B-cell activation, such as those recognized by the McAb CD21 and CD24, are negative or weakly expressed in a proportion of HCL cases [12].

The neoplastic cells in HCL express Ig in the membrane with high intensity with evidence of light-chain restriction. Concerning the Ig heavy-chain expression, there is a preferential use of certain Ig heavy chains in hairy cells. In the author and colleagues' and other investigators' experience, hairy cells express a high frequency IgG, and, particularly the IgG3 isotype [12,13]. This is in contrast to findings in other B-cell disorders in which cells express IgM/IgD more often; in addition, coexpression of several or even all four Ig heavy chains in HCL has been documented in a few cases [12,14–16]. This pattern of Ig heavy-chain expression in HCL contradicts that of the class-switching model that takes place in normal B-cell differentiation where switching from IgM/IgD to IgG or IgA occurs through a deletion of the constant region of the Ig gene. It was suggested that this error in class-switch is due to aberrations of the c-mu intron [15]. A recent study that focused on a small group of HCL cases in which cells expressed multiple Ig isotypes showed that the isotype switching events occur before deletional recombination, and suggested that this may be influenced by environmental factors [16]. Considering Ig light-chain expression, the proportion of κ- and λ-positive cases of HCL seems to be approximately equal [12]. Therefore, there is an increase in cases with λ light-chain expression over what is expected to be found in normal B cells (κ/λ ratio in normal B lymphocytes = 2) or even in the clonal B cells from other lymphoproliferative diseases, such as chronic lymphocytic leukemia (CLL) or prolymphocytic leukemia (PLL).

Hairy cells express several pan–B-cell markers, such as CD19, CD20, and CD37, and display a phenotypic profile that is different from that of CLL. In the scoring system that is used to differentiate CLL from other B-cell malignancies, HCL–like other non-CLL malignancies–has low scores that range from 1 to 0 in contrast to CLL in which scores range from 3 to 5 [17]. Hairy cells share features with some of the other B-cell leukemias with regards to the expression of CD5, CD23, and FMC7, however. In contrast to CLL and similar to B-cell PLL and B-cell lymphomas in leukemic phase, hairy cells are positive with the McAb FMC7, which identifies an epitope of the CD20 multi-meric complex [18]; the neoplastic cells express CD22 in the cell membrane strongly, whereas generally they are CD23 and CD5 negative. Unlike most of the other mature B-cell leukemias but like CLL, cells from two thirds of cases of HCL are negative with McAb's against CD79b, a marker that detects an epitope of the B-cell receptor β chain [12,19]. The reason for the absent or weak CD79b expression in HCL is unknown, but mutations or deletions of the CD79b gene have not been investigated in HCL as in CLL [20]. The latter studies might provide insights into the biology of this disease. Hairy cells do not express the antigen that is recognized by the McAb CD27, which is a marker that characteristically is present in memory B cells, in the minority of circulating normal marginal memory B cells, and in a wide range of other B-cell malignancies [21]. Other McAb's, such as CD38 and CD10, rarely are positive in hairy cells [22].

Cells in most cases of HCL are positive, with a variety of markers that are believed to be characteristic of this disease. These include CD11c, HC2 (non-clustered), CD103, and the α-chain of the interleukin (IL)-2 receptor; the last is recognized by the McAb's of the CD25 cluster [3,12,23,24]. It has been documented that serum levels of soluble IL-2 receptors (sCD25) correlate with disease activity or response to treatment; however, this serologic assay is not used routinely in clinical practice.

In addition, recent data showed that hairy cells express the α chain of the IL-3 receptor (CD123) [25]. CD123 is expressed in a variety of hemopoietic tumors, such as natural killer and dendritic cell malignancies, B-cell but not T-cell acute lymphoblastic leukemia, and acute myeloid leukemias; however, CD123 expression, with the exception of HCL, is extremely rare in mature B-cell disorders, including HCL-variant and splenic lymphoma with villous lymphocytes (SLVL) [25,26].

From the practical point of view, it is important to consider that none of the above markers is specific to HCL, and that some of them may be positive in cells from other B-cell disorders, including those with circulating blood villous cells (eg, SLVL or splenic marginal zone lymphoma [SMZL] and HCL-variant) [25,27]. Therefore, a composite phenotype that considers the expression of all or most of these antigens needs to be taken into account for a differential diagnosis. The author and colleagues documented that when four of these markers, such as CD11c, CD25, CD103, HC2, are compounded into a scoring system, the immunophenotypic profile of HCL is different from that seen in the HCL-variant and SLVL/SMZL [12,28]. This scoring system gives one point when the marker is positive and no point when the marker is negative; scores range from 4 (phenotype typical of HCL) to 0 (phenotype atypical for HCL). Their data showed that greater than 98% of cases of HCL have scores of 3 or 4, whereas low scores (0 or 1) are common in HCL-variant and SLVL. Because HC2 is not available commercially, the author and colleagues recently suggested that this marker should be substituted with CD123, because like HC2, it is generally negative in HCL-variant and SLVL/SMZL (Fig. 1) [25].

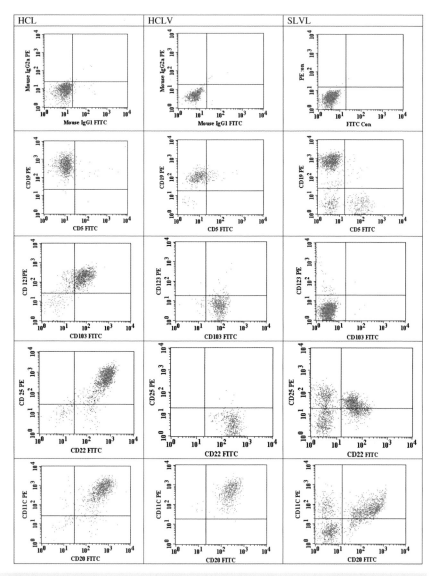

Fig. 1. Flow cytometry dot plots of cases of HCL (*left*), HCL-variant (HCLV; *middle*) and SLVL (*right*), which illustrate the characteristic immunophenotypic profiles of these diseases. In all three disorders the neoplastic cells are CD19+, CD20+, CD22++ (strong), and CD5−. HCL cells express CD25, CD11c, CD103, and CD123; HCL-variant cells are CD11c+, CD103+, but CD25− and CD123−; and the neoplastic cells in SLVL are CD11c+, CD25+, but CD103− and CD123− FITC, fluorescein conjugated; PE, phycoerytherine.

An important new finding relevant to the diagnosis of HCL was derived from gene expression profiling. This concerns the up-regulation of a gene, designated annexin A1, in the hairy cells [29]. Annexin A1 is involved in the phagocytosis pathway and in the regulation of cell signaling and proliferation. Immunohistochemistry using a McAb against annexin A1 (ANXA1) in a large number of samples from patients who had B-cell malignancies demonstrated the high sensitivity and specificity of this marker for HCL [29]. In this study, all cases of HCL were annexin A1 positive, whereas this molecule was not expressed in cells from the other B-cell diseases.

From a practical point of view and because in most patients there are few circulating hairy cells and the bone marrow aspirate is often dry-tap, immunohistochemistry applied in paraffin-embedded tissue sections with a panel of McAb's is important to establish the diagnosis. Among these, CD20, DBA44, and TRAP are the McAb's that are used on a routine diagnosis basis because all of them are strongly positive in HCL (Figs. 2–4). Although DAB44, CD20 and TRAP are not completely specific for the disease, because CD20 is a pan–B-cell marker and the more restricted DBA44 may be expressed in cells from other B-cell malignancies (eg, lymphoplasmacytic, marginal and mantle cell lymphomas) [30,31], the pattern of bone marrow infiltration and the cell morphology that is highlighted by the immunostaining helps to distinguish HCL from the other B-cell disorders. As outlined below, immunostaining with the McAb annexin A1 should provide useful diagnostic information because of the suggested specificity of this marker within the context of B-cell malignancies.

Other markers with potential diagnostic or biologic value in HCL include TIA-1, adhesion molecules, cyclin D1, and CD52.

TIA-1

This McAb identifies the granular content in a subset of cytotoxic CD8$^+$ T cells. Although not investigated extensively in HCL, a recent study showed that TIA-1 was expressed in one half (5/9) of cases of HCL that were analyzed; although TIA-1 lacks specificity, it may have a potential diagnostic value within the spectrum of B-cell malignancies. In this study, cells from most, if not all,

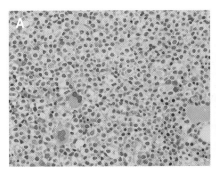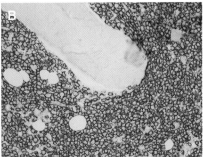

Fig. 2. (A) Bone marrow section from a patient who has hairy cell leukemia showing infiltration by hairy cells with the characteristic "fried egg" pattern. (B) Immunohistochemistry illustrating strong expression of CD20 in the hairy cells (immunoperoxidase technique).

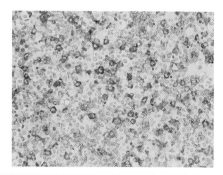

Fig. 3. Bone marrow section showing an interstitial infiltration by hairy cells highlighted by the immunostaining with the McAb DBA44 (immunoperoxidase technique).

B-cell disorders, except HCL, were TIA-1 negative [32]. Although further studies are needed to corroborate this, this finding is of interest because CD103, a marker that is expressed consistently in HCL and in certain T-cell lymphomas, also is positive characteristically on a subset of $CD8^+$ cytotoxic T cells [33].

Adhesion molecules

In most cases, hairy cells express a variety of adhesion receptors, such as the integrins CD18, CD49d, ICAM-1 (CD54), and the homing receptor CD44 [34]. Although there are some differences in the pattern of expression of these molecules in the various B-cell lymphoproliferative disorders, no unique adhesion phenotypic profile distinguishes HCL from other B-cell diseases. Whether expression of these adhesion molecules is related to a distinct pattern of homing of hairy cells (eg, a preferential spleen and abdominal nodal involvement without peripheral lymphadenopathy) is unknown. To this end, a study suggested that CD44 and hyaluronan interactions are relevant in the homing of hairy

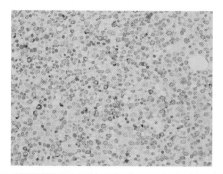

Fig. 4. Immunohistochemistry with the McAb anti-TRAP showing a dot/granular pattern of reactivity in scattered hairy cells (immunoperoxidase technique).

cells to the bone marrow and the hepatic portal tracts, but not to the spleen or hepatic sinusoids [35].

Cyclin D1

This cyclin is expressed in most cases of HCL and functions as a regulator of the cell cycle at the G1-S transition. The cyclin D1 is encoded by the bcl-1 gene and is mapped to chromosome 11q13. Overexpression of bcl-1/cyclin D1 is characteristic and is a hallmark of mantle cell lymphoma; however, it also can be up-regulated in some chronic lymphoid disorders, including HCL, few splenic non–mantle cell lymphomas, and multiple myeloma. Expression or up-regulation of the cyclin D1 has been documented in HCL by Northern and Western blots for m-RNA and protein expression, respectively, as well as by immunocytochemistry [36,37]. The overexpression of this cyclin in HCL does not seem to be associated with bcl-1 rearrangement or amplification of this gene, however. Thus, the mechanisms by which cyclin D1 is overexpressed in HCL seem to be different from those that take place in mantle cell lymphomas, and are unrelated to rearrangements or translocations of the bcl-1 locus.

CD52 expression

In addition to the strong expression of CD20 and CD22, hairy cells express CD52 with strong intensity [38]. Thus, Campath-1H, rituximab, and anti-CD22 McAb's, alone or in combination with purine analogs, are suitable to treat patients who have resistant disease.

Variant Form of Hairy Cell Leukemia

The immunophenotypic profile of cells in the HCL-variant is, as in typical HCL, different from CLL and also seems to correspond to that of a differentiated mature B cell; however, information is scanty concerning molecular studies that might support that the cells in HCL-variant are close to memory B cells. The neoplastic cells in this disease express a variety of pan-B markers, such as CD19, CD20, and CD22–the last with strong intensity–and, they often are positive with FMC7 but negative with McAb's against CD5 and CD23. The CLL scores are consistently low (<2). The CD24 and CD79b McAb's are positive in less than one third of cases [39,40], like in typical HCL. As in typical HCL, IgG is the most common Ig isotype chain that is expressed by the neoplastic cells. In the authors and colleagues' [39] experience, IgG, alone or in combination with other Ig heavy-chain isotypes, is found in more than half (56%) of cases. A minority of cases of HCL-variant does not express Ig in the membrane or in the cytoplasm; this feature is extremely infrequent in the clonal mature B-cell malignancies (leukemias and lymphomas), including normal and malignant plasma cells, which are cytoplasmic Ig positive. Regarding the Ig light-chain expression, there is a predominance of λ-positive versus κ-positive cases in the HCL-variant, and this is significantly higher than that seen in typical HCL and in other B-cell neoplasms. Thus, up to two thirds of cases of HCL-variant stain with anti-λ Ig chain. Unlike typical HCL, cells in the HCL-variant generally are CD25, HC2, and CD123 negative, whereas a substantial proportion of cases expresses CD11c and CD103 (see Fig. 1) [25,39,40]. In the scoring system for the diagnosis of HCL, the scores in the HCL-variant generally range from 0 to 2 [28]. Immunohistochemistry on tissue sections from bone marrow, spleen, or other organs demonstrates expression of CD20 and DBA44 in most cases [39]. The experience regarding expression of annexin A1 in HCL-variant is scanty. In the seminal report, only two cases that were described as HCL-variant seem to have been assessed, and both were negative [29]. Further studies in a larger number of cases of well-documented HCL-variant are needed to determine whether cells are annexin A1 positive.

In addition to the HCL-variant that was described in the Western countries, a variant form of HCL that seems to have some of the features of HCL-variant, such as high lymphocyte counts, lack of CD25 expression in the HCL-variant, and resistance to α-interferon, but having a similar histology to typical HCL, was described in Japan [41,42]. The relationship between these two variants is uncertain.

Markers for Detecting Residual Hairy Cell Leukemia

In addition to the diagnostic value of immunophenotyping, cell markers are useful for assessing response and detecting minimal residual disease (MRD) in patients who have HCL following therapy with the purine analogs 2′deoxycoformycin (pentostatin) and 2-chlorodeoxyadenosine (cladribine), or for monitoring disease status during these treatments. Residual disease in HCL can be investigated on paraffin-embedded bone marrow tissue sections with the McAb's DBA44 and CD20, or on mononuclear blood and bone marrow cells by triple- or quadruple-color flow cytometry using the panel of McAb's that is known to be expressed in HCL (eg, CD11c, CD25, CD103, CD123) [43–46]. The power of immunophenotyping for MRD detection was documented in some studies in which it was more sensitive than was polymerase chain reaction in the detection of residual hairy cells [45].

Overall, findings on MRD in HCL are variable as is their clinical significance. This may be due to the low recurrence rate of HCL in patients who achieved a complete remission as evaluated by standard criteria, and that relapses may become apparent after a long period of time. Therefore, long-term follow-up of these patients is required to conclude firmly on the clinical impact of detecting MRD in HCL. Nevertheless, some studies indicate that there is a trend for a higher probability of relapse in patients who have residual disease as detected by markers, than in those who have negative findings.

DIFFERENTIAL DIAGNOSIS

The differential diagnosis of typical HCL and HCL-variant arises with other B-cell lymphoproliferative disorders, particularly those evolving with splenomegaly or cytopenias (Table 1); T-cell large granular lymphocyte (LGL) leukemia; and a miscellaneous category, which includes mainly aplastic anemia, primary myelofibrosis, and mast cell diseases. In addition, typical HCL should

Table 1
Distinguishing features of splenomegalic mature B-cell disorders

	HCL	HCL-variant	SMZL/SLVL	B-PLL
WBC (>30 × 10⁶/l)	No	++	+	+++
Monocytopenia	yes	no	no	no
Palpable nodes	no	+	+	+
Morphology				
Cell size	medium	medium	small	medium
Cytoplasm	villous	villous	villous	regular
	abundant	abundant	small	small
Nucleolus	no	yes	no	yes
Immunophenotype				
CD11c	+++	+++	++	+
CD25	+++	neg	+	+
CD103	+++	++	neg	neg
CD123	+++	neg	neg	neg
CD24	++	+	+++	+++
CD79b	++	+	+++	+++
Histology				
BM	Spacing	Spacing	No spacing	No spacing
	Int + intras	Int + intras	nodular + intras	Often diffuse
Spleen	Red pulp	Red pulp	White pulp	White and
			(marginal zone)	red pulp

Abbreviations: +, positive in 10% to 30% of cases; ++, positive in 31% to 60% of cases; +++, positive in more than 60% of cases; int, interstitial; intras, intrasinusoidal; neg, positive in less than 10% of cases; WBC, white blood cell count.

be distinguished from the variant form because the clinical course and response to the purine analogs are significantly different [39].

The distinction between typical HCL and HCL-variant is based on the clinical features (normal monocyte count and high white blood cell count in the HCL-variant), morphology, and immunophenotype (HCL-variant cells generally are CD25 and CD123 negative) (Figs. 5 and 6). The pathology of the

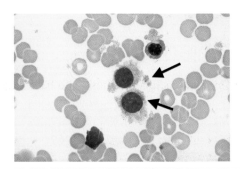

Fig. 5. May Grumwald Giemsa stained bone marrow smear from typical HCL showing an erythroblast and two lymphoid cells with abundant hairy cytoplasm (arrows).

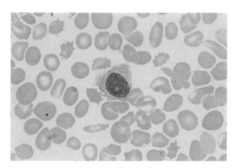

Fig. 6. Circulating cell from HCL-variant showing a round nucleus with prominent single nucleolus and a villous cytoplasm.

spleen and bone marrow is similar or identical in the two diseases; therefore, this investigation is not useful in the differential diagnosis. The differential diagnosis of typical HCL rarely arises with the other splenomegalic B-cell disorders, because the immunophenotype, morphology, and histology are unique to, and characteristic of, HCL.

Conversely, problems of differential diagnosis among HCL-variant, SLVL, and B-PLL do exist. There is overlapping on marker expression among these three conditions; nevertheless, a few differences can be exploited for the differential diagnosis. More than two thirds of cases of HCL-variant are negative with the McAb's CD24 and CD79b, whereas these two markers often are positive in SLVL/SMZL and B-PLL. In addition, and, in contrast to HCL-variant, CD103 is expressed rarely in SLVL/SMZL, whereas CD25 may be positive in up to one third of cases of SLVL/SMZL; generally, this marker is negative in HCL-variant. Conventional spleen histology helps to differentiate SLVL/SMZL (white pulp infiltration with expansion of the marginal zone) from HCL-variant (red pulp infiltration) The bone marrow histology also may be helpful, because although intrasinusoidal infiltration may be seen in SLVL and HCL-variant, nodular aggregates are not present in the HCL-variant. Rarely, the differential diagnosis of these conditions arises with mantle cell lymphoma. In such a case, morphology, histology, immunophenotype, and cytogenetics differentiate this lymphoma from HCL, the variant form, and SLVL.

A summary of the distinguishing features of the splenomegalic B-cell disorders is shown in Table 1.

The differential diagnosis of HCL with T-cell LGL leukemia arises in patients who have HCL who do not have peripheral blood involvement but a substantial proportion of circulating LGL, a feature that is not uncommon in HCL. The spleen histology in the two conditions shows a predominant infiltration of the red pulp; immunohistochemistry is unable to distinguish the two diseases.

A few patients who have HCL present with a hypoplastic bone marrow with mild hairy cell infiltration and severe cytopenias that mimic an aplastic anemia. Immunohistochemistry highlights the subtle hairy cell infiltrate, which allows it to be distinguished from aplastic anemia. Mast cell diseases may be confused with HCL because the pattern of involvement may be similar. Giemsa stain that shows metachromatic granules in the mast cells and immunohistochemistry distinguish HCL from mast cell diseases. Primary myelofibrosis can be distinguished from HCL by morphology and immunohistochemistry.

SUMMARY

HCL and HCL-variant cells have a distinct immunophenotype that seems to correspond to that of a mature activated memory B cell. Although the two diseases have similarities in histology and membrane marker expression, such as the selected Ig heavy-chain expression and the reactivity with certain B-cell activation markers (eg, CD103), there are differences in their clinical course, morphology, and immunophenotype. Immunophenotyping is an essential tool for the diagnosis of these two disorders, for monitoring and assessing response to therapy, and for distinguishing them from other B-cell malignancies.

Acknowledgments

The flow cytometry and histology illustrations were provided by Dr. Andrew Wotherspoon and Mr. Ricardo Morilla.

References

[1] Bouroncle BA, Wiseman BK, Doan CA. Leukemic reticuloendotheliosis. Blood 1958;13: 609–30.

[2] Foucar K, Catovsky D. Hairy cell leukaemia. In: Jaffe ES, Harris NL, Stein H, et al, editors. WHO classification of tumours of haematopoietic and lymphoid tissues. Lyon (France): IARC Press; 2001. p. 138–41.

[3] Korsmeyer SJ, Greene WC, Cossman J, et al. Rearrangement and expression of immunoglobulin genes and expression of Tac antigen in hairy cell leukemia. Proc Natl Acad Sci U S A 1983;80:4522–6.

[4] Cawley JC, Burns GF, Hayhoe FGJ. A chronic lymphoproliferative disorder with distinctive features: a distinct variant of hairy cell leukemia. Leuk Res 1980;4:547–59.

[5] Sainati L, Matutes E, Mulligan S, et al. A variant form of hairy cell leukemia resistant to alpha-interferon: clinical and phenotypic characteristics of 17 patients. Blood 1990;76:157–62.

[6] Zinzani PL, Lauria F, Buzzi M, et al. Hairy cell leukemia variant: a morphologic, immunologic and clinical study of 7 cases. Haematologica 1990;75:54–7.

[7] Yam LT, Li CY, Lam KW. Tartrate resistant acid phosphatase isoenzyme in the reticulum cells of leukaemic reticuloendotheliosis. N Engl J Med 1971;284:357–60.

[8] Drexler HG, Gignac SM. Characterisation and expression of tartrate-resistant acid phosphatase (TRAP) in hematopoietic cells. Leukaemia 1994;8:359–68.

[9] Hoyer JD, Li CY, Yam LT, et al. Immunohistochemical demonstration of acid phosphatase isoenzyme 5 (tartrate-resistant) in paraffin sections of hairy cell leukaemia and other hematologic disorders. Am J Clin Pathol 1997;108:308–15.

[10] Baso K, Liso A, Tiacci E, et al. Gene expression profiling of hairy cell leukaemia reveals a phenotype related to memory B-cells with altered expression of chemokine and adhesion receptors. J Exp Med 2004;199:59–68.

[11] Miranda RN, Cousar JB, Hammer RD, et al. Somatic mutation analysis of IGH variable regions reveal that tumor cells of most parafollicular (monocytoid) B-cell lymphoma, splenic marginal zone B-cell lymphoma and some hairy cell leukemia are composed of memory B lymphocytes. Hum Pathol 1999;30:306–12.

[12] Brito-Babapulle V, Matutes E, Catovsky D. Cytogenetics, molecular genetics and immunophenotyping in hairy cell leukaemia. In: Tallman MS, Polliack A, editors, Hairy cell

leukaemia. Advances in blood disorders, vol. 5. Amsterdam: Harwood Academic Publishers; 2000. p. 49–64.

[13] Kluin-Nelemans HC, Krouwels MM, Jansen JH, et al. Hairy cell leukemia preferentially expresses the IgG3 subclass. Blood 1990;75:972–5.

[14] Kinashi T, Godal T, Noma Y, et al. Human neoplastic B cells express more than two isotypes of immunoglobulins without deletion of heavy constant region genes. Genes Dev 1987;1: 465–70.

[15] Kayano H, Dyer MJS, Zani VJ, et al. Aberrant rearrangements within the immunoglobulin heavy chain locus in hairy cell leukemia. Leuk Lymphoma 1994;14(Suppl 1):41–7.

[16] Forconi F, Sahota SS, Raspadori D, et al. Hairy cell leukaemia: at a crossroad of somatic mutation and isotype switch. Blood 2004;104:3312–6.

[17] Matutes E, Owusu-Ankomah K, Morilla R, et al. The immunological profile of B-cell disorders and proposal of a scoring system for the diagnosis of CLL. Leukemia 1994;8:1640–5.

[18] Delgado J, Matutes E, Morilla A, et al. Diagnostic significance of CD20 and FMC7 expression in B-cell disorders. Am J Clin Pathol 2003;12:754–9.

[19] Zomas AP, Matutes E, Morilla R, et al. Expression of the immunoglobulin-associated protein B29 in B-cell disorders with the monoclonal antibody SN8 (CD79b). Leukemia 1996;10: 1966–70.

[20] Thompson AA, Talley JA, Do HN, et al. Aberrations of the B-cell receptor B29 (CD79b) gene in chronic lymphocytic leukemia. Blood 1997;90:1387–94.

[21] Forconi F, Raspadori D, Lenoci M, et al. Absence of surface CD27 distinguishes hairy cell leukaemia from other leukemic B-cell disorders. Haematologica 2005;90:266–8.

[22] Jasionowski TM, Hartung L, Greenwood JH, et al. Analysis of CD10$^+$ hairy cell leukaemia. Am J Clin Pathol 2003;120:228–35.

[23] Possnett DN, Chiorazzi N, Kunkel HG. Monoclonal antibodies reactive with hairy cell leukaemia. J Clin Invest 1982;70:254–61.

[24] Visser L, Shaw A, Slupsky J, et al. Monoclonal antibodies reactive with hairy cell leukaemia. Blood 1989;74:320–5.

[25] Del Giudice I, Matutes E, Morilla R, et al. The diagnostic value of CD123 in B-cell disorders with hairy or villous lymphocytes. Haematologica 2004;89:303–8.

[26] Munoz L, Nomdedeu JF, Lopez O, et al. Interleukin-3 receptor alpha chain (CD123) is widely expressed in hematologic malignancies. Haematologica 2001;86:1261–9.

[27] Matutes E, Morilla R, Owusu-Ankomah K, et al. The immunophenotype of splenic lymphoma with villous lymphocytes and its relevance to the differential diagnosis with other B-cell disorders. Blood 1994;83:1558–62.

[28] Matutes E, Morilla R, Owusu-Ankomah K, et al. The immunophenotype of hairy cell leukemia (HCL). Proposal for a scoring system to distinguish HCL from B-cell disorders with hairy or villous lymphocytes. Leuk Lymph 1994;14(Suppl 1):57–61.

[29] Falini B, Tiacci E, Liso A, et al. Simple diagnostic assay for hairy cell leukaemia by immunocytochemical detection of annexin A1 (Anxa1). Lancet 2004;363:1869–70.

[30] Salomon-Nguyen F, Valensi F, Troussard X, et al. The value of monoclonal antibody DBA44 in the diagnosis of B-lymphoid disorders. Leuk Res 1996;20:909–13.

[31] Ohsawa M, Kanno H, Machii T, et al. Immunoreactivity of neoplastic and non-neoplastic monocytoid B lymphocytes for DBA44 and other antibodies. J Clin Pathol 1994;47: 928–32.

[32] Mori N, Murakani YI, Shimada S, et al. TIA-1 expression in hairy cell leukemia. Mod Pathol 2004;17:840–6.

[33] Mulligan SP, Travade P, Matutes E, et al. Bly-7, a monoclonal antibody reactive with hairy cell leukemia, also defines an activation antigen on normal CD8$^+$ T cells. Blood 1990;76:959–64.

[34] Csanaky G, Matutes E, Vass JA, et al. Adhesion receptors on peripheral blood leukemic B cells. A comparative study on B cell chronic lymphocytic leukemia and related lymphoma/leukemias. Leukemia 1997;11:408–15.

[35] Aziz KA, Till KJ, Zuzel M, et al. Involvement of CD44-hyaluronan interaction in malignant cell homing and fibronectin synthesis in hairy cell leukemia. Blood 2000;96:3161–7.

[36] Bosch F, Campo E, Jares P, et al. Increased expression of the PRAD-1/CCND1 gene in hairy cell leukaemia. Br J Haematol 1995;91:1025–30.

[37] de Boer CJ, Kluin-Neleman SJC, Dreef E, et al. Involvement of CCND1 gene in hairy cell leukaemia. Ann Oncol 1996;7:251–6.

[38] Quigley MM, Bethel KJ, Sharpe RW, et al. CD52 expression in hairy cell leukemia. Am J Hematol 2003;74:227–30.

[39] Matutes E, Wotherspoon A, Brito-Babapulle V, et al. The natural history and clinico-pathological features of the variant form of hairy cell leukaemia. Leukemia 2001;15:184–6.

[40] Matutes E, Wotherspoon A, Catovsky D. The variant form of hairy cell leukaemia. Best Pract Res Clin Hematol 2003;16:41–56.

[41] Machii T, Tokumine Y, Inoue R, et al. Predominance of a distinct subtype of hairy cell leukemia in Japan. Leukemia 1993;7:181–6.

[42] Kondo H, Takeuchi H, Katayama I. Differentiating atypical HCL from HCL-Japanese variant. Leukemia 1996;10:384.

[43] Ellison DJ, Sharpe RW, Robbins BA, et al. Immunomorphologic analysis of bone marrow biopsies after treatment with 2-chlorodeoxyadenosine for hairy cell leukemia. Blood 1994;84:4310–5.

[44] Matutes E, Meeus P, McLennan K, et al. The significance of minimal residual disease in hairy cell leukaemia treated with deoxycoformycin: a long-term follow-up study. Br J Haematol 1997;98:375–83.

[45] Sausville JE, Salloum RG, Sorbara L, et al. Minimal residual disease detection in hairy cell leukemia. Comparison of flow cytometry immunophenotyping with clonal analysis using consensus primer polymerase chain reaction for the heavy chain gene. Am J Clin Pathol 2003;119:213–7.

[46] Wheaton S, Tallman MS, Hakimian D, et al. Minimal residual disease may predict bone marrow relapse in patients with hairy cell leukaemia treated with 2-chlorodeoxyadenosine. Blood 1996;87:1556–60.

Hematol Oncol Clin N Am 20 (2006) 1065–1073

HEMATOLOGY/ONCOLOGY CLINICS
OF NORTH AMERICA

Clinical Presentations and Complications of Hairy Cell Leukemia

Mark A. Hoffman, MD[a,b,*]

[a]Department of Medicine, Albert Einstein College of Medicine, 1300 Morris Park Avenue, Bronx, NY 10461, USA
[b]Division of Hematology-Oncology, Department of Medicine, Long Island Jewish Medical Center, 270-05 76th Avenue, New Hyde Park, NY 11040, USA

GENERAL CLINICAL PRESENTATION OF PATIENTS WHO HAVE HAIRY CELL LEUKEMIA

Bouroncle and colleagues [1] were the first to describe hairy cell leukemia (HCL) as a distinct clinicopathologic entity. At the time the illness was known as leukemic reticuloendotheliosis, based on an assumed origin from reticuloendothelial cells. The investigators described 26 patients who were seen over an 8-year period at Ohio State University. The male/female ratio was 4.2:1, with a range of 33–76. The most common presenting symptoms/signs were weakness and easy fatigability (46%), pain in the left upper quadrant due to splenomegaly (15%), bleeding manifestations (15%), in association with an infection (15%), and with infiltrative skin lesions (12%).

With regards to physical findings, the most common finding was splenomegaly, which was present in 96% of cases. In 14% of patients the spleen was enlarged moderately and in 42% it was enlarged markedly (defined as extending to the pelvic brim). Palpable hepatomegaly was seen in 58% of the cases. Lymphadenopathy was present in 35% of the patients; this particular aspect is addressed later in the article. Infiltrative skin lesions were seen in three patients in this group; cutaneous manifestations of HCL are rare (see later discussion).

With regards to the clinical course, infection was seen in 58% of patients at some time in their illness and was a common cause of death.

Hematologic observations revealed anemia in 77% of the patients. Most frequently, the anemia was believed be related to marrow infiltration and splenomegaly, but in six of the cases was "frankly hemolytic" based on reticulocytosis, hyperbilirubinemia, a positive Coombs test, and increased osmotic fragility. Leukopenia was seen in 58% of patients, with neutropenia in

*Division of Hematology-Oncology, Department of Medicine, Long Island Jewish Medical Center, 270-05 76th Avenue, New Hyde Park, NY 11040. E-mail address: mhoffman@lij.edu

0889-8588/06/$ – see front matter
doi:10.1016/j.hoc.2006.06.003

78% of cases. Marked thrombocytopenia ($<100,000/\mu L$) was seen in 46% of patients.

Autopsy of eight patients revealed liver, spleen, and lymph node involvement in all cases, but kidney, stomach, intestine, pancreas, and adrenal involvement also were seen, which attests to the systemic nature of the disease.

Bouroncle [2] subsequently published on 82 patients, including the original 26 cases. The overall male/female ratio was 4.5:1 and the median age was 55 years (range, 22–76 years). The most common presenting symptoms/signs were weakness and fatigue (51% of cases), concurrent infection (17%), left upper quadrant pain (14%), and hemorrhagic phenomena, such as ecchymoses, purpura, and epistaxis (9%). The disease was an incidental finding in 9% of cases. Splenomegaly was found in 93% of patients (marked in 53%); moderate hepatomegaly was seen in 43% and lymphadenopathy was seen in 23% ("discrete," measurements not given). Five patients (6%) had "skin infiltrations." Anemia was seen in 84% of patients, leukopenia was seen in 50%, and thrombocytopenia was seen in 58%. On autopsy material, spleen, lymph nodes, and liver were involved in most cases, with occasional involvement of lungs, kidney, pancreas, and adrenals.

Katayama and Finkel [3] published on 13 patients and reviewed the literature as of 1974. In their series, splenomegaly was omnipresent but lymphadenopathy was absent. They tabulated the findings in 98 patients who were described previously in the literature (including the original Bouroncle series). There was a marked male predominance, splenomegaly was almost universal, hepatomegaly was seen in one quarter to one half of cases, and lymphadenopathy was seen in 20% of the patients. Anemia and thrombocytopenia occurred in most cases, with leukopenia present in about half of the cases.

Subsequent series were published by Burke and colleagues [4] and Golomb and colleagues [5]. In Burke and colleagues' series of 21 patients, 19 had splenomegaly but only 4 had hepatomegaly and no patient had significant lymphadenopathy. In Golomb and colleagues' review of 71 cases, 83% had palpable splenomegaly, hepatomegaly (span >12 cm) was seen in 19%, and significant adenopathy (>3 cm) was seen in 10% (usually in only one site).

In 1994, Frassoldati and colleagues [6] for the Italian Cooperative Group for Hairy Cell Leukemia analyzed a series of 725 patients that was accrued to an HCL registry over a 25-year period. The male/female ratio, as in the older series, was approximately 4:1, and the mean age at diagnosis was 54 years. They analyzed the clinical presentation at diagnosis for patients who were diagnosed before 1975, between 1976 and 1980, between 1981 and 1984, between 1985 and 1987, and from 1988 to 1990. There was a progressive decline in mean spleen size over the different time periods; patients with no palpable spleen or mildly palpable spleen represented 30.2% of patients before 1975 and 52% of the patients after 1985. The number of patients with a hemoglobin level of less than 8.5 g/dL at diagnosis decreased from 40% before 1975 to 24.7% after 1985. The reason for the earlier disease burden at diagnosis was believed to be the result of improved diagnostic techniques [6].

OTHER LABORATORY FINDINGS

As above, some patients in the original Bouroncle and colleagues [1] series were described as having a hemolytic component to the anemia, with mention of a positive Coombs test. Nonetheless, autoimmune hemolytic anemia and auto-immune thrombocytopenic purpura, which are not uncommon in B-cell chronic lymphocytic leukemia [7], have been reported rarely in patients who have HCL [8–10].

Janckila and colleagues [11] examined the blood of 40 patients who had HCL, and found a marked reduction of monocyte numbers; this was a persistent observation over time in individual patients. Along with other cytopenias, monocyte counts normalize with cladribine therapy [12].

As reviewed by Cohen and colleagues [13], monoclonal immunoglobulins are found uncommonly in HCL. Even when found, the paraprotein is of small quantity and likely is incidental.

Juliusson and colleagues [14] found hypocholesterolemia in most of their 61 patients. The hypocholesterolemia was not due to increased low-density lipoprotein receptor uptake by the hairy cells. Cholesterol levels increased after therapy, which is consistent with a disease-related variable [14].

HAIRY CELL LEUKEMIA VARIANT

HCL variant is distinguished from HCL by the cell morphology and different immunophenotypic profile [15,16]. There is a difference in the clinical manifestations as well. There is only a slight male predominance. As in HCL, splenomegaly is the major clinical finding. As opposed to the usual laboratory features of typical HCL, lymphocytosis is found frequently and there is no monocytopenia [15,16].

COMPLICATIONS AND UNUSUAL MANIFESTATIONS OF HAIRY CELL LEUKEMIA

Infection

Before the advent of effective therapy for HCL, infections were the major cause of death [1,6]. Patients who have HCL are predisposed to infections because of neutropenia, impaired neutrophil microbicidal function [17], monocytopenia [11], monocyte dysfunction [18], and marked deficiency in circulating dendritic cells [19]. With these defects, there is a resultant susceptibility to bacterial infections, as well as to infections that usually are contained by cell-mediated immunity. The use of chemotherapy and corticosteroids in the period before splenectomy, as well as splenectomy itself, also contributed to the risk for infection.

Golomb and Hadad [20] analyzed the infectious complications of 127 patients between 1974 and 1982. Eighty-seven patients had infections: 47 were documented (culture-positive) infections and 40 were culture-negative infections. The infection-related mortality was 62% (29/47). Infections were pyogenic (bacterial) and nonpyogenic. Of the nonpyogenic infections, 8 were due to *Aspergillus fumigatus*, 5 were due to *Mycobacterium kansaii*, 3 were due to *Pneumocystis carinii*, and 1 was due to *M tuberculosis*. The 40 patients who did not have infectious episodes had an excellent survival, which established infection as the major cause of death in HCL.

Bennett and colleagues [21] corroborated the association of HCL and serious infection with atypical mycobacteria. Disseminated atypical mycobacterial infections (six with *M kansaii*, two with *M avium-intracellulare*, and one with *M cheloneii*) were seen in 9 of 186 patients. This topic since has been reviewed briefly by Thaker and colleagues [22].

In addition to the typical pathogenic bacteria, there have been reports of infection by *Legionella* [23], *Pasteurella* [24], *Capnoctophaga* [25], *Histoplasma* [26], *Cryptococcus* [27], *Mucormycosis* [28], and *Zygomycosis* [29].

With the advent of interferon therapy and the induction of disease remission, infection as a cause of death declined [6]. In the era of purine analog therapy, infectious complications have become rare. In an extended follow-up (at least 7 years) of 207 patients who were treated with cladribine, only 6 patients had died and there was only one documented death from infection [30].

Splenic Rupture

Despite the massive splenomegaly that is seen in most patients who have HCL, spontaneous rupture of the spleen is rare. It can be the presenting feature in HCL, or it may occur in the course of the disease [31,32].

Massive Adenopathy

Mercieca and colleagues [33] reported on 12 patients who had massive abdominal adenopathy. Eight of the 12 had longstanding HCL (median, 10 years from diagnosis). The adenopathy was ascertained by CT scanning for various symptoms. A confluent mass of retroperitoneal lymph nodes—centered around the celiac axis and upper para-aortic and retro-pancreatic areas—was found in all patients. Biopsy of these nodes in five cases revealed the typical small lymphoid cells, but there also were admixed larger, more immature cells with prominent nucleoli. Immunophenotyping of the nodal biopsy in one patient was typical of HCL.

Although peripheral adenopathy is uncommon in HCL, the prevalence of significant internal adenopathy is unknown. Based on this series, it likely is a late-onset phenomenon that is associated with histologic transformation.

Skin Manifestations

Finan and colleagues [34] reported a case of leukemia cutis in a patient who had HCL, and reviewed the cutaneous findings that were seen at the time of diagnosis or during the disease course of 113 patients who were seen at the Mayo Clinic. Ecchymotic lesions were seen in 28% of cases and petechiae were seen in 19%. The most common category of skin lesion was infection (herpetic, cellulites abscess, pyoderma, dermatophytosis). There was only the single case of leukemia cutis.

Carsuzaa and colleagues [35] reviewed the cutaneous findings in 47 patients in two French hospitals over a 10-year period. Fifty-eight percent of the lesions were of infectious origin. Most these infections were of bacterial origin, and manifested as cellulitis or abscess. In addition to bacterial, viral, and fungal infections, skin lesions may be due to atypical mycobacteria [36,37]. Isolated reports of leukemia cutis have been published [34,38,39].

Pyoderma gangrenosum has been seen in HCL [40,41], and Sweet's syndrome (neutrophilic dermatosis) also has been reported [42,43]. Finally, leukocytoclastic vasculitis may be seen as part of the spectrum of vasculitis in HCL (see later discussion) [44].

Skeletal Involvement

Lembersky and colleagues [45] reviewed the records of 267 patients who had HCL at the University of Chicago and identified 8 patients with bone involvement. The lesions were lytic and primarily involved the proximal femur. The lesions were discovered on imaging that was performed to assess pain in the areas of involvement. One patient had a pathologic fracture. Local radiotherapy was effective treatment in all instances. Weh and colleagues [46] identified 5 patients among 150 patients who were seen over 19 years. The lesions involved the femoral head in 4 of the 5 patients and there was one pathologic fracture. Snell and colleagues [47] reported a patient who had a pathologic femoral fracture and reviewed the literature as of 1999. The lesions were lytic and femoral neck or head involvement was seen in 77% of cases. Other sites were skull, vertebrae, ribs, humerus, pelvis, tibia, and fibulae.

Neurologic Manifestations

There are isolated reports of leukemic meningitis in HCL [48,49]. The patient who was reported by Wolfe and colleagues [48] responded to intrathecal chemotherapy and whole brain radiotherapy. One patient developed bilateral facial nerve palsy that was due to infiltration of both auditory channels by HCL [50]. This patient had been diagnosed 36 years earlier and had been treated with splenectomy and chemotherapy. Treatment with cladribine led to almost complete resolution of the patient's symptoms.

Rheumatologic Diseases/Vasculitis

There has been a significant association between HCL and vasculitic syndromes, most recently reviewed by Hasler and colleagues [51]. They classified the types of vasculitis into three distinct groups: (1) polyarteritis nodosa, as diagnosed by typical aneurysms on angiography; (2) leukocytoclastic vasculitis, ascertained by skin biopsy; and (3) direct invasion of vessel walls by hairy cells. Of the cases of polyarteritis nodosa, most occurred after splenectomy, and hepatitis B surface antigen was positive in 3 of 12 cases. Leukocytoclastic vasculitis often appeared before HCL, and often was preceded by infection. The mechanisms underlying the association between HCL and polyarteritis nodosa/leukocytoclastic vasculitis have not been elucidated, but may be related to hepatitis B infection, delayed clearance of immune complexes after splenectomy, or an autoantibody against an antigen (HC1) that is expressed on hairy cells and endothelial cells [52]. That vasculitis may be related directly to HCL is supported by the response of the vasculitis to effective HCL therapy [53–55].

Inflammatory arthritis or arthralgias may occur in the course of HCL [56,57]. As outlined in a case report/literature review by Vernhes and colleagues [58], the arthritis is polyarticular and may have features of rheumatoid arthritis in half of cases. Arthritis may be caused directly by synovial involvement by HCL [59].

OTHER RARE DISEASE PRESENTATIONS/ASSOCIATIONS

Bouroncle [60] reported a case of gastric infiltration and two cases with ascites with hairy cells in the ascetic fluid. Schofield and colleagues [61] reported a patient who presented with nephrotic syndrome and HCL. Associations with scleroderma [62,63] and sarcoidosis [64] have been reported. One case of retinal vasculitis/uveitis has been published [65].

SECOND MALIGNANCIES

An issue of considerable controversy has been whether there is an increased risk for second malignancies in patients who have HCL ,and if so, is it attributable to a specific therapy (eg, splenectomy, interferon) as opposed to an intrinsic aspect of the disease.

Among recent series, Au and colleagues compared the relative risk for second malignancies, as compared with a control population, in 117 patients in British Columbia between 1976 and 1996. The prevalence of second malignancies was 22%, and the relative rate of second malignancies was 2.6 times that of the matched population [66]. Kurzrock and colleagues [67], in a study of 350 patients from 1968 to 1995, found a 7.4% risk for second malignancies and no increased risk over a control population. Flinn and colleagues [68] analyzed 241 patients who were treated with pentostatin and found no increased incidence of second malignancies. Goodman and colleagues [30] found a twofold increased risk in 207 patients who were treated with cladribine. The largest patient population (1022 patients) was studied by the Italian Cooperative Study Group. There was no overall increased risk for second malignancies; however, there was an increased incidence of non-Hodgkin's lymphoma [69]. None of the studies in patients who were treated with different modalities was able to discern an association between treatment type (splenectomy, interferon, pentostatin) and incidence of second malignancies. In addition, with regards to the type of second malignancy, there was no consistent pattern across these studies. In summary, if there is an increased risk for second malignancy in HCL, it likely is small, and there is inconsistent evidence for increased risk for any one malignancy.

SUMMARY

HCL typically presents in middle-aged men, and is characterized by splenomegaly and cytopenias. Hepatomegaly may be present, but it usually is not a salient feature. Peripheral adenopathy is uncommon. Other organ manifestations occur, but are unusual. Patients are now presenting with a less tumor burden, as a result of earlier diagnosis. Leukocytosis/lymphocytosis should suggest HCL variant.

Infectious complications, which were common in the past and the major cause of death, have become rare in the era of purine analog therapy. Whether there is a true increased risk for second malignancies remains controversial.

References

[1] Bouroncle B, Wiseman BK, Doan C. Leukemic reticuloendotheliosis. Blood 1958;13(7): 609–30.

[2] Bouroncle B. Leukemic reticuloendotheliosis (hairy cell leukemia). Blood 1979;53(3): 412–33.

[3] Katayama I, Finkel H. Leukemic reticuloendotheliosis. A clinicopathologic study with review of the literature. Am J Med 1974;57:115–25.

[4] Burke JS, Byrne GE, Rappaport H. Hairy cell leukemia (leukemic reticuloendotheliosis). Cancer 1974;33(5):1399–410.

[5] Golomb HM, Catovsky D, Golde DW. Hairy cell leukemia. A clinical review based on 71 cases. Ann Intern Med 1978;89:677–83.

[6] Frassoldati A, Lamparelli T, Federico M, et al. Hairy cell leukemia: a clinical review based on 725 cases of the Italian Cooperative Group (ICGHCL). Leuk Lymphoma 1994;13:307–16.

[7] Domingo A, Crespo N, deSavillo A, et al. Hairy cell leukemia and autoimmune hemolytic anemia. Leukemia 1992;6(6):606–7.

[8] Moullet I, Salles G, Dumontete C, et al. Severe autoimmune thrombocytopenic purpura and haemolytic anemia in a hairy-cell leukemia patient. Eur J Hematol 1995;54:127–9.

[9] Mainwaring CJ, Walewska R, Snowden J, et al. Fatal cold anti-I autoimmune hemolytic anemia complicating hairy cell leukemia. Br J Haematol 2000;109:641–3.

[10] Kipps TJ, Carsons DA. Autoantibodies in chronic lymphocytic leukemia and related systemic autoimmune disease. Blood 1993;81:2475–87.

[11] Janckila AJ, Wallace JH, Yam LT. Generalized monocyte deficiency in leukemic reticuloendotheliosis. Scand J Hematol 1982;29(2):153–60.

[12] Juliusson G, Lilliemark J. Rapid recovery from cytopenias in hairy cell leukemia after treatment with 2-chloro-2'-deoxyadenosine (CdA): relation to opportunistic infections. Blood 1992;79:888–94.

[13] Cohen O, Mor F, Beigel Y, et al. The significance of paraproteinemia in hairy cell leukemia: case report and review of the literature. Haematologica 1990;75(2):179–81.

[14] Juliusson G, Vitols S, Liliemark J. Disease related hypocholesterolemia in patients with hairy cell leukemia. Cancer 1995;76:423–8.

[15] Matutes E, Wotherspoon A, Brito-Babapulle V, et al. The natural history and clinico-pathological features of the variant form of hairy cell leukemia. Leukemia 2001;15:184–93.

[16] Matutes E, Wotherspoon A, Catovsky D. The variant form of hairy-cell leukemia. Best Pract Res Clin Hematol 2003;16(1):41–56.

[17] Child JA, Cawley JC, Martin S, et al. Microbicidal function of the neutrophils in hairy cell leukemia. Acta Haematol 1979;62(4):191–8.

[18] Nielsen H, Bangsborg J, Rechnitzer C, et al. Defective monocyte function in Legionnaire's disease complicating hairy cell leukemia. Acta Med Scand 1986;220(4):381–3.

[19] Bourguin-Plonquet A, Rouard H, Roudot-Thoraval F, et al. Severe decrease in peripheral blood dendritic cells in hairy cell leukemia. Br J Haematol 2002;116:595–7.

[20] Golomb HM, Hadad LJ. Infectious complications in 127 patients with hairy cell leukemia. Am J Hematol 1984;16:393–401.

[21] Bennett C, Vardiman J, Golomb H. Disseminated atypical mycobacterial infection in patients with hairy cell leukemia. Am J Med 1986;80(5):891–6.

[22] Thaker H, Neilly IJ, Saunders PG, et al. Remember mycobacterial disease in hairy cell leukemia (HCL). J Infect 2001;42(3):213–4.

[23] Fang GD, Stout JE, Yu VL, et al. Community-acquired pneumonia caused by *Legionella dumoffii* in a patient with hairy cell leukemia. Infection 1990;18(6):383–5.

[24] Athar MK, Karim MS, Mannam S, et al. Fatal *Pasteurella* sepsis and hairy cell leukemia. Am J Hematol 2003;72(4):285.

[25] Hartley JW, Martin ED, Gothard WP, et al. Fulminant *Capnocytophaga canomorus* (DF2) septicaemia and diffuse intravascular coagulation in hairy cell leukemia with splenectomy. J Infect 1994;29(2):229–30.

[26] Weeks E, Jones CM, Guinee V, et al. Histoplasmosis in hairy cell leukemia. Case report and review of the literature. Ann Hematol 1992;65:138–42.

[27] Audeh YM, Gruszecki AC, Cherrington A, et al. Hairy cell leukemia with concurrent cryptococcus infection. Am J Hematol 2003;72:223–4.

[28] Bennett CL, Westbrook CA, Gruber B, et al. Hairy cell leukemia and mucormycosis. Am J Med 1986;81:1065–7.

[29] Ma B, Seymour JF, Januszewicz H, et al. Cure of pulmonary *Rhizomucor pusillis* infection in a patient with hairy cell leukemia: role of liposomal amphotericin B and GM-CSF. Leuk Lymphoma 2001;42(6):1393–9.

[30] Goodman GR, Burian C, Koziol JA, et al. Extended follow-up of patients with hairy cell leukemia after treatment with cladribine. J Clin Oncol 2003;21(5):891–6.

[31] Bouroncle B. Unusual presentations and complications of hairy cell leukemia. Leukemia 1987;4:288–93.

[32] Keidan AJ, Liu Yin JA, Gordon-Smith EC. Uncommon complications of hairy cell leukemia. Br J Haematol 1984;57(1):176–7.

[33] Mercieca J, Matutes E, Moskovic E, et al. Massive adenopathy in hairy cell leukemia: a report of 12 cases. Br J Haematol 1992;82:547–54.

[34] Finan MC, Su WP, Chin-Yang L. Cutaneous findings in hairy cell leukemia. J Am Acad Dermatol 1984;11:788–97.

[35] Carsuzaa F, Pierre C, Viala JJ. Cutaneous findings in hairy cell leukemia. Review of 84 cases. Nouv Rev Fr Hematol 1993;35:541–3.

[36] Castor B, Juhlin I, Henriques B. Septic cutaneous lesions caused by Mycobacterium malmoense in a patient with hairy cell leukemia. Eur J Clin Microbiol Infect Dis 1994;13(2):145–8.

[37] Raanani P, Thaler M, Keller N, et al. Skin lesions in a patient with hairy cell leukemia. Postgrad Med J 1997;73(860):375–7.

[38] Lawrence D, Sun NCJ, Mena R, et al. Cutaneous lesions in hairy-cell leukemia. Arch Dermatol 1983;119:322–5.

[39] Bilsland D, Shahriari S, Douglas WS, et al. Transient leukemia cutis in hairy-cell leukemia. Clin Exp Dermatol 1991;16(3):207–9.

[40] Rustin MH, Staughton RC, Coomes EN. Hairy cell leukemia and pyoderma gangrenosum. J Am Acad Dermatol 1985;13:300–2.

[41] Cartwright PH, Rowell NR. Hairy cell leukemia presenting with pyoderma gangrenosum. Clin Exp Dermatol 1987;12(6):451–2.

[42] Gisser SO. Acute febrile neutrophilic dermatosis (Sweet's syndrome) in a patient with hairy cell leukemia. Am J Dermatopathol 1983;5:283–8.

[43] Fischer G, Commens C, Bradstock K. Sweet's syndrome in hairy cell leukemia. J Am Acad Dermatol 1989;21:573–4.

[44] Spann CR, Callen JP, Yam LT, et al. Cutaneous leucocytoclastic vasculitis complicating hairy cell leukemia (leukemic reticuloendotheliosis). Arch Dermatol 1986;122:1057–9.

[45] Lembersky BC, Ratain MJ, Golomb HM. Skeletal complications in hairy cell leukemia: diagnosis and therapy. J Clin Oncol 1988;6(8):1280–4.

[46] Weh HJ, Katz M, Bray B, et al. Lesions osseouses au cours des leucemies a tricholeucocytes [Bone lesions in hairy cell leukemia]. Nouv Presse Med 1979;8(27):2253–4 [in French].

[47] Snell KS, O'Brien MM, Sendelbach K, et al. Pathologic fracture occurring 22 years after diagnosis of hairy cell leukemia: case report and literature review. West J Med 1999;170: 172–4.

[48] Wolfe DW, Scopelliti JA, Boselli BD. Leukemic meningitis in a patient with hairy cell leukemia. Cancer 1984;54(6):1085–7.

[49] Navarrete D, Bodega E. Leukemic meningitis in a patient with hairy cell leukemia. Nouv Rev Fr Hematol 1987;29(4):247–9.

[50] Ferrari J, Lang W, Thurnher S, et al. Bilateral facial palsy as first indication of relapsing hairy cell leukemia after 36 years. Neurology 2004;63:399–400.

[51] Hasler P, Kistler H, Gerber H. Vasculitis in hairy cell leukemia. Semin Arthritis Rheum 1995;25(2):134–42.

[52] Posnett DN, Marboe CC, Knowles DM, et al. A membrane antigen selectively present on hairy cell leukemia cells, endothelial cells, and epidermal basal cells. J Immunol 1984; 132(6):2700–2.

[53] Gomez-Almaguer D, Herrera-Garza JL, Garcia-Guajardo BM, et al. Vasculitis in hairy cell leukemia: rapid response to interferon alpha. Am J Hematol 1989;30:261–2.

[54] Carpenter M, West SG. Polyarteritis nodosa in hairy cell leukemia; treatment with interferon-α. J Rheumatol 1994;21:1150–2.

[55] Seshadri P, Hadges S, Cropper T. Acute necrotising vasculitis in hairy cell leukemia-rapid response to cladribine: case report and a brief review of the literature. Leuk Res 2000;24(9):791–3.

[56] Westbrook CA, Golde DW. Autoimmune disease in hairy cell leukemia: clinical syndromes and treatment. Br J Haematol 1985;61:349–56.

[57] Zervas J, Vayopoulos G, Kaklamanis G, et al. Hairy cell leukemia-associated polyarthritis: a report of two cases. Br J Rheumatol 1991;30(2):157–8.

[58] Vernhes JP, Schaeverbeke T, Fach J, et al. Chronic immunity driven polyarthritis in hairy cell leukemia. Rev Rhum 1997;64(10):578–81.

[59] Sattar MA, Cawley MI. Arthritis associated with hairy cell leukemia. Ann Rheum Dis 1982;41(3):289–91.

[60] Bouroncle BA. Unusual presentations and complications of hairy cell leukemia. Leukemia 1987;1(4):288–93.

[61] Schofield KP, Vites N, Geary CG, et al. Nephrotic syndrome and hairy cell leukemia. Br J Haematol 1985;60(2):389–90.

[62] Cavallero GB, Bonferroni M, Gallamini A, et al. Scleroderma and hairy cell leukemia. Eur J Haematol 1994;52:189–90.

[63] Blanche P, Bachmeyer C, Mikdame M, et al. Scleroderma, polymyositis and hairy cell leukemia. J Rheumatol 1995;22:1384–5.

[64] Schiller G, Said G, Pal S. Hairy cell leukemia and sarcoidosis: a case report and review of the literature. Leukemia 2003;17(10):2057–9.

[65] Di Maria A, Redaelli C, Canevari A, et al. Unilateral retinal vasculitis associated with hairy cell leukemia: immunogenetic study. Ophthalmologica 1998;212:355–7.

[66] Au WY, Klasa RJ, Gallagher R, et al. Second malignancies in patients with hairy cell leukemia: a 20 year experience. Blood 1998;92(4):1160–4.

[67] Kurzrock R, Strom SS, Estey E, et al. Second cancer risk in hairy cell leukemia: analysis of 350 patients. J Clin Oncol 1997;15(5):1803–10.

[68] Flinn IW, Kopecky KJ, Foucar MK, et al. Long term followup of remission duration, mortality and second malignancies in hairy cell leukemia patients treated with pentostatin. Blood 2000;96(9):2981–6.

[69] Federico M, Zinzani P, Frassoldati A, et al. Risk of second cancer in patients with hairy cell leukemia: long-term follow-up. J Clin Oncol 2002;20(3):638–46.

Hematol Oncol Clin N Am 20 (2006) 1075–1086

HEMATOLOGY/ONCOLOGY CLINICS
OF NORTH AMERICA

SEVIER
UNDERS

Splenectomy, Interferon, and Treatments of Historical Interest in Hairy Cell Leukemia

Thomas M. Habermann, MD

Department of Hematology, Mayo Clinic College of Medicine, 200 First Street,
SW Rochester, MN 55905, USA

Hairy cell leukemia (HCL) is an uncommon leukemia. It was described first by Bertha Bouroncle and colleagues in 1958 [1]. After Hodgkin lymphoma, HCL has been a model for incorporating and understanding the clinical interventions of surgery, chemotherapy, biologic response modifiers, purine nucleoside analogs, and monoclonal antibody therapy. Advances in treatment, all of which were empiric at the time, preceded advancements in understanding the biology of the disease. The history of therapeutic intervention has been characterized by empiric interventions without scientific bench research applied to a disease that did not have good outcomes or therapeutic interventions. Such approaches have changed the natural history of this disease and opened doors for other diseases. Over time, the definitions of response evolved into modern response definitions. This article focuses on treatments of historical interest, observation, splenectomy, and the interferons.

TREATMENTS OF HISTORICAL INTEREST
The treatments of historical interest include

> Leukapheresis
> Lithium
> Androgens: halotestin, oxymethalone
> Single-agent alkylator chemotherapy: chlorambucil
> Combination chemotherapy
> Bone marrow transplantation
> Corticosteroids
> Radiation therapy
> High-dose methotrexate

These interventions are not used in HCL and are not incorporated into the management of this disease.

E-mail address: habermann.thomas@mayo.edu

0889-8588/06/$ – see front matter
doi:10.1016/j.hoc.2006.06.006

Leukapheresis

Therapeutic leukapheresis was introduced in 1965 [2]. This therapeutic intervention was used in the leukemic phase of hairy cell disease [3,4]. This only resulted in a transient decrease in the peripheral blood hairy cell count with no long-term improvement [5]. There was no impact on the bone marrow pattern or other peripheral blood counts.

Lithium

Lithium was used in the treatment of HCL [6]. There seemed to mild benefit for the leukopenia, but the toxicities were significant.

Androgens

Halotestin, 10 mg three times per day, or oxymetholone, 150 mg four times per day, was recommended for patients who were refractory to chlorambucil [7–9]. Long-term responses were documented in three of six cases [8].

Chlorambucil

At one time chlorambucil was the treatment of choice in HCL [10]; however, the response types and rates were low and the impact on the bone marrow was minimal. A dosage of 4 mg/d orally for at least 6 months initially was the treatment of choice in leukemic and leukopenic relapses after splenectomy [10]. Chlorambucil resulted in a decrease in the white blood cell count to less than 10,000 cells/μL in patients in the leukemic phase, and most patients showed some increase in platelet counts and hematocrits. In leukopenic patients, the neutropenia and leukopenia did not improve, and the risk for infection remained increased; however, there were changes in the hemoglobin and platelet counts. The bone marrow in most patients demonstrated a decreased cellularity and increase in normal marrow elements, but did not normalization in responders. These responses were, at best, minor by the standard chemotherapy response criteria. Myelodysplastic syndromes were reported with the use of this alkylator agent therapeutic intervention [11]. Other complications included infections. The survival after observation, splenectomy, and chlorambucil was reported to be 68% at 5 years in a series of 65 patients [12].

Combination Chemotherapy

Systemic chemotherapy has been incorporated without success in this disease [13]. In addition, it resulted in the prolonged exacerbation of the neutropenia and thrombocytopenia. CHOP (cyclophosphamide, doxorubicin, vincristine, and prednisone) was a more common regimen [14]. The regimen was not efficacious in HCL [15]. Combination chemotherapy resulted in prolonged cytopenias, life-threatening infections, and intensive supportive care that included transfusions and remissions that lasted less than 1 year. In cases of transformation to diffuse large B-cell non-Hodgkin lymphoma (DLBCL), CHOP has been used as the treatment of choice, followed by peripheral blood stem cell transplantation [16,17]. In patients who have undergone a transformation to DLBCL, rituximab in combination with CHOP is the treatment of choice [18,19].

Bone Marrow Transplantation
An identical twin went into a complete remission following allogeneic transplantation after induction with busulfan and cyclophosphamide followed by total body irradiation, with normal blood counts and no hairy cells in the bone marrow at 4 years [20]. The patient was disease-free at least 15 years after the transplant from an identical twin brother [21]. At this time, allogeneic transplantation should be limited to eligible patients who have failed nucleoside analog therapy and other interventions.

Corticosteroids
A systemic vasculitis may occur in HCL. Joint involvement and fevers are characteristic. High-dose steroids have been advocated, especially after splenectomy, but have predisposed patients to opportunistic infections [22,23]. The purine nucleoside analogs have supplanted this approach.

Radiation Therapy
Lytic lesions of the femur with potential fractures have been reported in HCL [24]. Radiation therapy has been used as an intervention in this clinical manifestation of the disease. A major role for splenic irradiation was never established. Low-dose splenic irradiation has been advocated as a therapeutic option for the rare elderly patient who has massive splenomegaly [25].

High-Dose Methotrexate
High-dose methotrexate (2 g/m^2), followed by leucovorin rescue, was administered every 4 to 6 weeks [26]. Five patients had improvement in peripheral blood counts without significant myelosuppression, and in two patients the response was of 14 and 44 months' duration.

ALTERNATIVE APPROACHES TO THE PRESENT STANDARD OF CARE
Alternative approaches to the standard of care, 2-chlorodeoxyadenosine, include observation, splenectomy, interferon-α2a, and interferon-α2b. The indications for these therapeutic interventions include minimal disease, age, associated comorbidities, accompanying life-threatening infection, socioeconomic factors, and other unusual circumstances.

Observation
Efficacious therapeutic interventions have narrowed observation remarkably as an approach. It was suggested that 10% of patients did not need treatment [27]. Golomb [28] recommended observation in patients who were more elderly and had minimally palpable or nonpalpable spleens, and an absolute granulocyte count of 1000/μL or greater.

Patients who have minimal bone marrow interstitial hairy cell involvement, a minimally palpable or nonpalpable spleen, an absolute neutrophil count of greater than 1500/μL, hemoglobin greater than 12 g/dL, and platelet count greater than 100,000/μL are potential candidates for initial observation. Goodman [29] noted that watchful waiting is appropriate for asymptomatic patients who have HCL in whom significant cytopenias are absent because early treatment has not been of benefit to survival or response.

Splenectomy

Routine splenectomy was the standard of care for years before 1984 and the introduction of recombinant interferon followed by the purine nucleoside analogs 2-deoxycoformycin and 2-chlorodeoxyadenosine. Initially, splenomegaly was reported to occur at presentation or during the course of the disease in approximately 90% of patients [30,31]. This provided the rationale for splenectomy. No randomized controlled studies were performed. This therapeutic approach did not affect the bone marrow infiltration or pattern but did target the spleen, which is a major site of hairy cell proliferation.

The interpretation of the results of splenectomy is complex because standard response criteria, which are now incorporated into the response criteria in malignant disease, were not incorporated in HCL response criteria in splenectomy reports—presumably because splenectomy had no impact on the bone marrow. The definition of Catovsky [32] was implemented most commonly. Complete response (CR) was defined as a hemoglobin greater than 11 g/dL, absolute neutrophil count greater than 1000/μL, and a platelet count of greater than 100,000/μL. A partial response (PR) is the same degree of improvement in only one or two of these or improvement in all three, but less than the stated cutoffs. At best, these criteria would meet minor response criteria in interferon and nucleoside analog treatment trials. There was no provision for hairy cells in the peripheral blood.

With the above response criteria there are eight reports to review [8,12,21,33–37]. The CR and PR rates ranged from 60% to 100% (ie, 60%, 100%, 97%, 100%, 61%, 88%, 86%, and 62%, respectively). The only reported predictor of response was the hairy cell index that was reported by Golomb and Vardiman [12]. The hairy cell index was defined as the bone marrow cellularity expressed as a fraction multiplied by the fraction of hairy cells in the bone marrow, which results in a number between 0 and 1. An index of greater than 0.7 did not have a good response to splenectomy. Patients with spleens that were less than 4 cm below the costal margin only had improved hemoglobin if there was significant anemia before splenectomy [33].

Survival data in patients who underwent a splenectomy are complex and difficult to interpret. Patient populations are not comparable, the indications for splenectomy were variable, the timing of the splenectomy was variable, the data are predominantly retrospective, and the populations were selected for each management strategy for variable reasons. Jansen and colleagues [38] reported a median survival of 30 to 36 months and no difference with no splenectomy (55%) or splenectomy (75%) at 4 years. In 1981, Jansen and Hermans [35] reported a 48-month median survival, with a 38% survival at 5 years without splenectomy versus a 55% survival after splenectomy. Flandrin and colleagues [36] reported a statistical difference at 5 years after splenectomy (60%) versus 42% with no splenectomy. Damasio and colleagues [39] reported a median survival of 33 months in splenectomized patients and 27 months for nonsplenectomized patients.

Biologic observations back up the clinical observations that the spleen and bone marrow are the primary sites with some patients having hepatomegaly. This provides a biologic rationale for why surgical extirpation of the spleen removes a significant bulk disease. Hairy cells accumulate in the red pulp of the spleen because of the interaction of the functionally active integrin receptor, $\alpha_4\beta_1$, on hairy cells and vascular cell adhesion molecule-1, which is expressed in splenic endothelial cells, splenic stroma, bone marrow stroma, and hepatic endothelial cells, but not other endothelial cells [40]. Pseudosinuses–spaces that are filled with red blood cells lined by hairy cells rather than endothelial cells–also contribute to splenomegaly [41]. Consequently, 15% to 48% of the red blood cell mass has been reported to be in the spleen [42].

Splenectomy is not incorporated into the up-front management of the patient who has HCL. The treatment of choice, 2-chlorodeoxyadenosine, results in resolution of even massive splenomegaly as does deoxycoformycin and the recombinant interferons. Asplenic patients who present with fever should be treated with empiric antibiotics with appropriate spectrum coverage.

Interferon

Interferon was the first biologic response modifier to be approved by the U.S. Food and Drug Administration (FDA). The first report of activity was a landmark paper in 1984 by Quesada and colleagues [43]. Seven patients were treated with 3 million units (MU) of purified leukocyte interferon-α; three patients were reported to have a CR, and four patients were reported to have a PR with maintained remissions of 6 to 10 months' duration. The interferon-α class was the major group of interferons that was evaluated in HCL. Natural interferon-α, recombinant interferon-β, and recombinant interferon-γ were reported [43–45]; however, interferon-β and -γ did not have the efficacy in small numbers of patients [44,45]. A trial of human lymphoblastoid interferon-α, 3 MU daily for 5.7 months followed by 3 MU/m^2 weekly, reported a CR rate of 24%, a PR rate of 56%, and an overall survival of 85% at 58 months [46].

Two recombinant interferon-α drugs were developed, evaluated, and approved by the FDA in 1986: interferon-α2a (Roferon-A, Hoffmann-LaRoche, Inc., Nutley, New Jersey) and interferon-α2b (Intron-A, Schering-Plough Corp., Kenilworth, New Jersey) which differed by only one amino acid. Interferon improved peripheral blood counts, reduced spleen size, and reduced the bone marrow hairy cell infiltrate. For the first time, the response criteria included true complete remissions (ie, no morphologic evidence of disease). It was common to have patients on the hospital services who expired, something that is now uncommon.

Quesada and colleagues [47] reported on 30 patients who were treated at a single institution with recombinant interferon-α2a. Thirty percent (9) of patients were reported to be in CR and 56% (17) were reported to be in PR, and all had improvement or normalization of their peripheral blood counts. It was at about this time that the response criteria were developed for HCL that eventually were incorporated into the National Cancer Institute (NCI)-sponsored intergroup trial that evaluated recombinant interferon-α2a and 2-chlorodeoxyadenosine (deoxycoformycin). A CR was defined as a normalization of the peripheral blood counts (hemoglobin $\geq$12 g/dL, absolute neutrophil count $\geq$1.5 × 10^9/L, platelet count >100 × 10^9/L, and no circulating hairy cells), no organomegaly (splenomegaly and hepatomegaly), and an absence of hairy cells in the bone marrow. A PR included the same complete blood count parameters and less than 5% circulating hairy cells with a reduction in the hairy cell infiltrate by 50% or greater and a reduction in organomegaly by greater than 50%.

Subsequent trials unfolded rapidly nationally and internationally. In a multi-institution trial, 64 patients—61 with previous splenectomy and 31 with other previous treatment—were treated with interferon-α2b, 2 MU/m^2 subcutaneously three times per week, with a CR in 5% and a PR in 70% [48]. In a single-institution phase II study, recombinant interferon-α2a, 2 MU/m^2 three times per week for 1 year, and a CR defined as less than 5% hairy cells in the bone marrow resulted in a CR rate of 13% and the PR rate of 62%, with a median progression-free survival (PFS)/failure-free survival (FFS) of 25.4 months and an overall survival of 91% at 4 years [49]. The Cancer and Leukemia Group B reported on the long-term results on 55 patients who were treated with recombinant interferon-α2b, 2 MU/m^2 three times per week for 1 year. The CR rate was 24%, the PR rate was 49%, the PFS/FFS was 18 months, and the overall survival was 83% at 6 years [50]. In a trial at Memorial Sloan-Kettering Cancer Center, there were CRs in 35 patients, 69% PRs, and the median PFS/FFS was 10 months (range, 0.5–25 months) [51]. Smith and colleagues [52] reported a 2% CR rate and 74% PR rate in 56 patients who were treated with recombinant interferon-α, 3 MU daily for 6 months followed by three times per week for 6 to 60 months.

As the results of these trials were unfolding, and as it was evident that patients who had advanced disease were responding, data were brought together for FDA approval. Early on, it became apparent the bone marrow patterns were changing, transfusion requirements were going away, that patients were not having infectious complications, and that patients were no longer being hospitalized [53].

Treatment with interferon-α resulted in partial remissions that ranged from 69% to 87% [47–52]. The responses predominantly were partial remissions. There did not seem to be a major advantage between recombinant interferon-αa or recombinant interferon-α2b. There was significant activity in patients who had been treated previously with other modalities. Responses occurred in patients with or without a spleen. The initial response was a decrease in the peripheral blood hairy cells in the first week, an increase in the platelet count within 2 months, followed by increases in the hemoglobin in 4 months and in the white blood cell count within a median of 5 months [54,55]. Monocytopenia, a hallmark of the disease, also improved significantly in responders. Most patients had residual hairy cells and bone marrow fibrosis [54–56]. Over time, no modification in dose or schedule seemed to be more advantageous. Lower dosages were efficacious and were a change from the maximal tolerable dose schedules that were used in other diseases at the time.

One small prospective controlled trial randomized previously untreated patients to recombinant interferon-α or splenectomy [57]. The response rate was higher in the group that received recombinant interferon-α, and the median time to treatment failure was 18 months in the group that received interferon and 1 month in the group that underwent splenectomy.

The NCI convened a group to establish an intergroup trial of recombinant interferon-α versus pentostatin because of the comparative efficacy and safety of both agents. This was one of the first times that the NCI convened a group of investigators to plan and carry out studies in a specific disease entity and with specific agents. The initial results and long-term follow-up have been reported [58,59]. Patients were randomized to receive interferon-α2a, 3×10^6 U subcutaneously three times per week, or pentostatin, 4 mg/m^2 intravenously every 2 weeks. As anticipated, 79% of the patients in the arm that received interferon and 80% of the patients in the arm that received pentostatin were men. Among the patients who received interferon, 17 of 159 (11%) achieved a complete remission and 43 (27%) achieved a partial remission. In contrast, 117 of 154 patients (76%) who were treated with pentostatin achieved a complete remission and 4 (3%) achieved a partial remission. Response rates were significantly higher with pentostatin ($P = .0001$), relapse-free survival was significantly longer with pentostatin ($P = .0001$), and myelosuppression was more frequent with pentostatin ($P = .013$). Eighty-seven patients crossed over after failure on interferon. Twelve of the 17 patients who were treated with interferon relapsed between 9 and 27 months. The relapse-free survival did not differ significantly between those who received pentostatin as initial induction compared with those who crossed over from interferon therapy, with the 10-year estimate of survival of 67% at initial induction and 69% in the crossover population [59]. Grade 4 myelosuppression occurred in 9 of 158 (6%) patients who were treated with interferon and 22 of 154 (14%) patients who were treated with pentostatin ($P = .013$). There were fewer suspected infections during the induction phase with interferon (56 of 159; 35%) than with pentostatin (82 of 154, 53%; $P = .002$). Fourteen percent of patients who received interferon and 27% of patients who received pentostatin were treated with systemic antibiotic therapy.

In a randomized trial of splenectomized patients, there also was a longer duration of response with pentostatin [60]. Three patients who relapsed after cladribine responded to interferon-α [61].

The FDA approved the two interferons. The recommended dosage of interferon-α2b (Intron-A) is 2 MU/m^2 subcutaneously three times per week for 6 to 12 months. The recommended dosage of interferon-α2a (Roferon) is 3 MU subcutaneously three times per week for 12 months as per the randomized study. Higher dosages were associated with more toxicity and not with more efficacy [62]. Longer duration of therapy with maintenance dosages, 1 MU three times a week or 3 MU weekly, prolonged the response duration and maintained durable responses [52,63,64]. After an initial response in 76% (40/53) of patients, 32 patients were treated with maintenance interferon-α, 3 MU three times per week for a median of 5 years; 60% of patients sustained their initial response and 13% demonstrated progressive disease [52]. In a trial that randomized patients to observation or maintenance interferon-α (1 MU three times per week), 66% (37/56) of patients in the observation arm relapsed compared with 0% (0/28) of patients in the maintenance treatment arm at a median follow-up of 30 months [63].

The dosages that are incorporated in the treatment of HCL are tolerated well overall, but there are toxicities. Patients developed a tachyphylaxis to the flu-like symptoms of fevers and chills after 1 to 4 weeks [44–58]. Tylenol or non-steroidal anti-inflammatory agents are effective in managing these toxicities. Fatigue is the most common side effect. Nonsteroidal anti-inflammatory agents do not alter fatigue. Anorexia is more common than is vomiting or diarrhea. Depression and mood changes may occur at the standard HCL dosages. Neurologic toxicities include peripheral neuropathy, somnolence, lethargy, dizziness, confusion, and impaired mental status. Cardiovascular toxicities include atrial arrhythmia, sinus tachycardia, and hypotension. Other toxicities include rash at the injection site, small joint arthritis, hepatitis, alopecia, hypertrichosis, and decreased libido [63]. The white blood cell count and hemoglobin levels characteristically decrease during the first month of therapy. Mild elevation in liver function studies occurs. Exacerbation of a pre-existing autoimmune disease or the development of a new autoimmune disorder has been reported [65]. Although initially controversial, two large series did not show an increased incidence of second malignancies [59,66].

Neutralizing antibodies with recombinant interferon-α2b were low, but up to one third of patients developed a positive titer neutralizing interferon antibody with recombinant interferon-α2a [51,67,68]. Follow-up and further studies suggest that the antibodies are transient and that most patients become antibody negative after a median follow-up of 14.5 months [69].

The mechanism of action of interferon is unknown. Hairy cells express the interferon-α receptor [70]. Interferon-α functions as a cytostatic agent in HCL. Therefore, the primary mechanism of action is the induction of hairy cell differentiation toward a stage that is less responsive to growth stimulation. which results in inhibition of hairy cell proliferation [71]. Interferon induces hematopoietic growth factors within the leukemic cells by priming the production of endogenous interferon [72].

Interferon Combination Therapy

Combination therapy was evaluated with 3 months of interferon followed by pentostatin (2'-chlorodeoxyadenosine) [73]. These data demonstrated that an initial course of α-interferon may improve the peripheral blood counts. This is not recommended routinely. In the event of a fever of undetermined etiology or a known atypical mycobacterial infection, initial treatment with interferon-α2a or -α2b to improve the immune function—as manifested by neutropenia, lymphocyte population aberrations, and monocytopenia—should be considered. Initially, there were two reports of significant improvement in immune reconstitution and survival in the setting of *Mycobacterium avium* infection.

SUMMARY

The evolution and "lessons learned" for therapeutic options and approaches in HCL, which subsequently evolved into the adenosine deaminase inhibitors as the treatment of choice, has been intriguing [74–77]. The contributions to patient care and individual patient lives have been remarkable [78]. Observation, splenectomy, and recombinant interferon are potential therapeutic alternatives in select patients as initial therapy, and as therapeutic alternatives in the 10% of patients who have progressive disease after the purine nucleoside analogs.

References

[1] Bouroncle BA, Wiseman BK, Doan CA. Leukemic reticuloendotheliosis. Blood 1958;13: 609–30.

[2] Freireich EJ, Judson G, Levin RH. Separation and collection of leukocytes. Cancer Res 1965;25:1516–20.

[3] Fay JW, Moore JO, Logue GL, et al. Leukapheresis therapy of leukemic reticuloendotheliosis (hairy cell leukemia). Blood 1979;54:747–9.

[4] Mielke CH Jr, Dobbs CE, Winkler CF, et al. Therapeutic leukapheresis in hairy cell leukemia. Arch Intern Med 1982;142:700–2.

[5] Golomb HM, Kraut EH, Oviatt DL, et al. Absence of prolonged benefit of leukapheresis in hairy cell leukemia. Am J Hematol 1983;14:49–56.

[6] Blum SF. Lithium in hairy cell leukemia. N Engl J Med 1980;303:464–5.

[7] Lusch CJ, Ramsey HE, Katayama I. Leukemic reticuloendotheliosis. Report of a case with peripheral blood remission on androgen therapy. Cancer 1978;41:1964–6.

[8] Magee M, McKenzie S, Filippa DA, et al. Hairy cell leukemia: durability of response to splenectomy in 26 patients and treatment of relapse with androgens in six patients. Cancer 1985;56:2557–62.

[9] Keffer SE, Westring DW, Lee AC, et al. A case of leukemic reticuloendotheliosis responding to oxymethalone. Cancer 1982;50:396–400.

[10] Golomb HM. Progress report on chlorambucil therapy in post-splenectomy patients with progressive hairy cell leukemia. Blood 1981;57:464–7.

[11] Albain KS, Le Beau MM, Vardiman JW, et al. Development of a dysmyelopoietic syndrome in a hairy cell leukemia patient treated with chlorambucil: cytogenetic and morphologic evaluation. Cancer Genet Cytogenet 1983;8:107–15.

[12] Golomb HM, Vardiman JW. Response to splenectomy in 65 patients with hairy cell leukemia: an evaluation of spleen weight and bone marrow involvement. Blood 1983;61: 349–52.

[13] Calvo F, Castiagne S, Sigaux F, et al. Intensive chemotherapy in patients with aggressive disease. Blood 1985;65:115–9.

[14] Fisher RI, Gaynor ER, Dahlberg S, et al. Comparison of a standard regimen (CHOP) with three intensive chemotherapy regimens for advanced non-Hodgkin's lymphoma. N Engl J Med 1993;328:1002–6.

[15] Cold S, Brincker H. Chemotherapy of progressive hairy cell leukemia. Eur J Haematol 1987;38:251–5.

[16] Downing JR, Grossi CE, Smedberg CT, et al. Diffuse large cell lymphoma in a patient with hairy cell leukemia: immunoglobulin gene analysis reveals separate clonal origins. Blood 1986;67:739–44.

[17] Bolwell B, Kalaycio M, Andresen S, et al. Autologous peripheral blood progenitor cell transplantation for transformed diffuse large-cell lymphoma. Clin Lymphoma 2000;1(3): 226–31; discussion 232–3.

[18] Coiffier B, Lepage E, Briere J, et al. CHOP chemotherapy plus rituximab compared with CHOP alone in elderly patients with diffuse large B-cell lymphoma. N Engl J Med 2002;346:235–42.

[19] Habermann TM, Weller E, Morrison VA. Rituximab CHOP versus CHOP with or without maintenance rituximab in patients 60 years of age or older with diffuse large B-cell lymphoma (DLBCL). J Clin Oncol 2006;24:3121–7.

[20] Cheever MA, Fefer A, Greenberg PD, et al. Treatment of hairy cell leukemia with chemoradiotherapy and identical-twin bone marrow transplantation. N Engl J Med 1982;307: 479–81.

[21] Bouroncle B. Thirty-five years in the progress of hairy cell leukemia. Leuk Lymphoma 1994;14(Suppl 1):1–12.

[22] Golddert JJ, Neeje JR, Smith FS, et al. Polyarteritis nodosa, hairy cell leukemia, and splenosis. Am J Med 1981;71:323–6.

[23] Elkon KB, Hughes GRV, Catovsky D, et al. Hairy cell leukemia with polyarteritis nodosa. Lancet 1979;2:280–2.

[24] Demanes DJ, Lane N, Beckstead JH, et al. Bone involvement in hairy-cell leukemia. Cancer 1982;49:1697–702.

[25] Nishii K, Katayama N, Maeda H, et al. Successful treatment with low dose splenic irradiation for massive splenomegaly in an elderly patient with hairy cell leukemia. Eur J Haematol 2001;67:255–7.

[26] Joosten P, Hagenbeek A, Lowenberg B, et al. High-dose methotrexate with leucovorin rescue: effectiveness in relapsed hairy cell leukemia. Blood 1985;66:241–2.

[27] Postnett DN, Chiorazzi N, Kunkel HG. Monoclonal antibodies with specificity for hairy cell leukemia cells. J Clin Invest 1982;70:254–61.

[28] Golomb HM. Hairy cell leukemia: lessons learned in twenty-five years. J Clin Oncol 1983;1:652–6.

[29] Goodman GR, Bethel KJ, Saven A. Hairy cell leukemia: an update. Curr Opin Hematol 2003;10(4):258–66.

[30] Katayama I, Finkel HE. Leukemic reticuloendotheliosis. A clinicopathologic study with review of the literature. Am J Med 1974;57:115–25.

[31] Golomb HM. Hairy cell leukemia: an unusual lymphoproliferative disease. A study of 24 patients. Cancer 1978;42:946–56.

[32] Catovsky D. Hairy cell leukemia and prolymphocytic leukemia. Clin Haematol 1977;6: 245–68.

[33] Jansen J, Hermans J. Clinical staging system for hairy-cell leukemia. Blood 1982;60: 571–6.

[34] Mintz U, Golomb H. Splenectomy as initial therapy in twenty-six patients with leukemic reticuloendotheliosis (hairy cell leukemia). Ca Res 1979;39:2366–70.

[35] Jansen J, Hermans J. Splenectomy in hairy cell leukemia: a retrospective multicenter analysis. Cancer 1981;47:2066–76.

[36] Flandrin G, Sigaux F, Sebhoun G, et al. Hairy cell leukemia: clinical presentation and follow-up of 211 patients. Sem Oncol 1984;11(Suppl 2):458–71.

[37] van Norman A, Nagorney D, Martin K, et al. Splenectomy for hairy cell leukemia: a clinical review of 63 patients. Cancer 1986;57:644–8.

[38] Jansen J, Hermans J, Remme J, et al. Hairy cell leukemia: clinical features and effects of splenectomy. Scand J Haematol 1978;21:60–71.

[39] Damasio E, Spriano M, Repetto M, et al. Hairy cell leukemia: a retrospective study of 235 cases by the Italian Cooperative Group (ICG HCL) according to Jansen's clinical staging system. Acta Haematol 1984;72:326–34.

[40] Vincent AM, Burthem J, Brew R, et al. Endothelial interaction of hairy cells: the importance of $\alpha 4\beta 1$ in the unusual tissue distribution of the disorder. Blood 1996;88: 3945–52.

[41] Nanba K, Jaffe E, Soban E, et al. Hairy cell leukemia: enzyme histochemical characterization, with special reference to splenic stromal changes. Cancer 1977;39:2323–36.

[42] Lewis S, Catovsky D, Hows J, et al. Splenic red cell pooling in hairy cell leukemia. Br J Haematol 1976;35:351–7.

[43] Quesada JR, Reuben J, Manning JT, et al. Alpha interferon for induction of remission in hairy cell leukemia. N Engl J Med 1984;310:15–8.

[44] Glapsy JA, Marcus SG, Amersley J, et al. Recombinant beta-serine-interferon in hairy cell leukemia compared prospectively with results with recombinant alpha-interferon. Cancer 1989;64:409–13.

[45] Quesada JR, Alexanian R, Kursrock R, et al. Recombinant interferon gamma in hairy cell leukemia, multiple myeloma, and Waldenstrom's macroglobulinemia. Am J Hematol 1988; 29:1–4.

[46] Capnist G, Federico M, Chisesi T, et al. Long term results of interferon treatment in hairy cell leukemia. Italian Cooperaptive Group of Hairy Cell Leukemia (ICGHCL). Leuk Lymphoma 1994;14:457–64.

[47] Quesada JR, Hersh EM, Manning J, et al. Treatment of hairy cell leukemia with recombinant alpha-interferon. Blood 1986;68:493–7.

[48] Golomb HM, Jacobs A, Fefer A, et al. Alpha-2 interferon therapy for hairy cell leukemia: a multicenter study of 64 patients. J Clin Oncol 1986;4:900–5.

[49] Retain MJ, Golomb HM, Vardiman JW, et al. Relapse after interferon-α-2b for hairy cell leukemia: analysis of prognostic variables. J Clin Oncol 1988;6:1714–21.

[50] Rai KR, Davey F, Peterson B, et al. Recombinant alpha-2b-interferon in therapy of previously untreated hairy cell leukemia: long-term follow-up result of study by Cancer and Leukemia Group B. Leukemia 1995;9:1116–20.

[51] Berman E, Heller G, Kempin S, et al. Incidence and response and long-term follow-up in patients with hairy cell leukemia treated with recombinant-α-interferon-2b. Blood 1990; 75:839–45.

[52] Smith JW II, Longo DL, Urba JW, et al. Prolonged continuous treatment of hairy cell leukemia with recombinant interferon-α-2a. Blood 1991;78:1664–71.

[53] Habermann TM, Hoagland HC, Chang M, et al. A phase II trial of alpha recombinant leukocyte interferon (alpha-R-IFN) in hairy cell leukemia in patients with advanced disease: marked improvement in bone marrow, periheral blood parameters, and decreased red blood cell transfusions. Blood Suppl 1983;66:200a.

[54] Bardawil RG, Groves C, Ratain MJ, et al. Changes in peripheral blood and bone marrow specimens following therapy with recombinant alpha2 interferon for hairy cell leukemia. Am J Clin Pathol 1986;85:194–201.

[55] Flandrin G, Sigaux F, Castaigne S, et al. Treatment of hairy cell leukemia with recombinant alpha interferon: 1. Quantitative study of bone marrow changes during the first months of treatment. Blood 1986;67(3):817–20.

[56] Ratain MJ, Golomb HM, Vardiman JW, et al. Durability of responses to interferon alpha-2b in advanced hairy cell leukemia. Blood 1987;69:872–7.

[57] Smally RV, Connors J, Tuttle RJ, et al. Splenectomy vs. alpha interferon: a randomized study in patients with hairy cell leukemia. Am J Hematol 1992;41:13–8.

[58] Grever M, Kopecky K, Foucar KM, et al. Randomized comparison of pentostatin versus interferon alfa-2a in previously untreated patients with hairy cell leukemia: an intergroup study. J Clin Orthod 1995;13:974–82.

[59] Flinn IW, Kopecky KJ, Foucar MK, et al. Long-term follow-up of remission duration, mortality and second malignancies in hairy cell leukemia patients treated with pentostatin. Blood 2000;96:2981–6.

[60] Rai KR. Comparison of pentostatin and alpha interferon in splenectomized patients with active hairy cell leukemia: an intergroup study. Cancer and Leukemia Group B and South-West Oncology Group. Leuk Lymphoma 1994;14(Suppl 1):107–8.

[61] Seymour JF, Estey EH, Keating MJ, et al. Response to interferon-α in patients with hairy cell leukemia after treatment with 2-chlorodeoxyadenosine. Leukemia 1995;9:929–32.

[62] Quesada JR, Talpaz M, Rios A, et al. Clinical toxicity of interferons in cancer patients: a review. J Clin Oncol 1986;4(2):234–43.

[63] Troussard X, Flandrin G. Hairy cell leukemia. An update on a cohort of 93 patients in a single institution. Effects of interferon in patients relapsing after splenectomy and in patients relapsing after splenectomy and in patients with or without maintenance treatment. Leuk Lymphoma 1994;14S:99–105.

[64] Speilberger RT, Mick R, Retain MJ, et al. Interferon treatment for hairy cell leukemia. An update on a cohort of 69 patients treated from 1983 to 1986. Leuk Lymphoma 1994;14S: 89–93.

[65] Conlon KC, Urba WJ, Smith JW II, et al. Exacerbation of symptoms of autoimmune disease in patients receiving alpha-interferon therapy. Cancer 1990;65:2237–42.

[66] Rawson R, A'hern R, Catovsky D. Second malignancy in hairy cell leukemia: no evidence of increased incidence after treatment with interferon-α. Leuk Lymphoma 1996;22:103–6.

[67] Spiegel R, Spicehandler JR, Jacobs SL, et al. Low incidence of serum neutralizing factors in patients receiving recombinant alfa-2b interferon (Intron A). Am J Med 1986;80:223–8.

[68] Spiegel R, Jacobs SL, Treuhaft MW. Anti-interferon antibodies to interferon-α2b: results of comparative assays and clinical perspective. J Interferon Res 1989;9(S):17–24.

[69] Steis RG, Smith JW II, Urba WJ, et al. Loss of interferon antibodies during prolonged continuous interferon-alpha 2a therapy in hairy cell leukemia. Blood 1991;77:792–8.

[70] Platanias LC, Preffer LM, Barton KP, et al. Expression of the IFN alpha receptor in hairy cell leukemia. Br J Haematol 1992;82:541–6.

[71] Vedantham S, Gamliel H, Golomb HM. Mechanisms of interferon action in hairy cell leukemia: a model of effective cancer biotherapy. Cancer Res 1992;52:1056–66.

[72] Shehata M, Sehwarzmier JD, Nguyen ST, et al. Reconstitution of endogenous interferon a by recombinant interferon in hairy cell leukemia. Cancer Res 2000;60:5420–6.

[73] Habermann TM, Anderson JW, Cassileth PA, et al. Sequential administration of alpha recombinant interferon followed by deoxycoformycin in the treatment of hairy cell leukemia. Brit J Haematol 1992;80:466–71.

[74] Golomb HM, Catovsky D, Golde DW. Hairy cell leukemia: a clinical review based on 71 cases. Ann Intern Med 1978;89:677–83.

[75] Westbrook CA, Groopman JE, Golde DW. Hairy cell leukemia: disease pattern and prognosis. Cancer 1984;54:500–6.

[76] Golde DW. Therapy of hairy cell leukemia. N Engl J Med 1982;307:495–6.

[77] Turner A, Kjeldsberg CR. Hairy cell leukemia: a review. Medicine 1978;57:477–99.

[78] Kurland G. My own medicine: a doctor's life as a patient. New York: Times Books, Henry Holt and Company; 2002.

HEMATOLOGY/ONCOLOGY CLINICS
OF NORTH AMERICA

SEVIER
UNDERS

Purine Analogues: Rationale for Development, Mechanisms of Action, and Pharmacokinetics in Hairy Cell Leukemia

Gunnar Juliusson, MD[a,b,*], Jan Liliemark, MD[c]

[a]Stem Cell Center, BMC B10, Lund University, SE-221 84 Lund, Sweden
[b]Department of Hematology EA12, Lund University Hospital, SE-221 85 Lund, Sweden
[c]Medical Products Agency, PO Box 26, SE-75103, Uppsala, Sweden

DEVELOPMENT OF NUCLEOSIDE ANALOGS FOR CANCER TREATMENT

Nucleosides are important compounds in human physiology and are precursors for DNA and RNA. Natural nucleosides are activated by intracellular phosphorylation by deoxycytidine kinase (dCK), and this step may be reversed by nucleotidases. Another important step for deactivation is deamination through adenosine deaminase (ADA). Nucleoside analogs may be metabolized similarly to their natural counterparts, incorporated into DNA or RNA, and, thereby, cause metabolic disturbances, apoptosis, and cell death. Therefore, nucleoside analogs were developed starting in the late 1940s as potential anticancer agents. Mercaptopurine was the first compound that was studied successfully [1,2], and was followed by cytosine arabinoside (Fig. 1) [3,4]; these remain important drugs in the treatment of acute leukemia.

In the 1960s, adenine-based nucleosides were developed, including adenosine arabinose (ara-A). Ara-A was cytotoxic in vitro, but rapid deamination led to deactivation. This problem could be solved by adding pentostatin (deoxycoformycin), which is a tight inhibitor of ADA, the key enzyme for deactivation. Thus, Ara-A plus deoxycoformycin act synergistically, whereas treatment with deoxycoformycin by itself leads to the accumulation of natural nucleotides in cells with a high dCK activity. Another possibility for the improvement of ara-A was the introduction of a halogen in the 2-position of the adenine, which blocks the binding of ADA, and, thereby, protects the compound from deactivation through deamination. The latter option was used for the development of F-ara-A (9-beta-D-arabinofuranosyl-2-fluoroadenine) [5,6], the active metabolite of fludarabine (see Fig. 1), and several other compounds.

*Corresponding author. Stem Cell Center, BMC B10, Lund University, SE-221 84 Lund, Sweden. *E-mail address:* Gunnar.Juliusson@med.lu.se (G. Juliusson).

0889-8588/06/$ – see front matter
doi:10.1016/j.hoc.2006.06.007

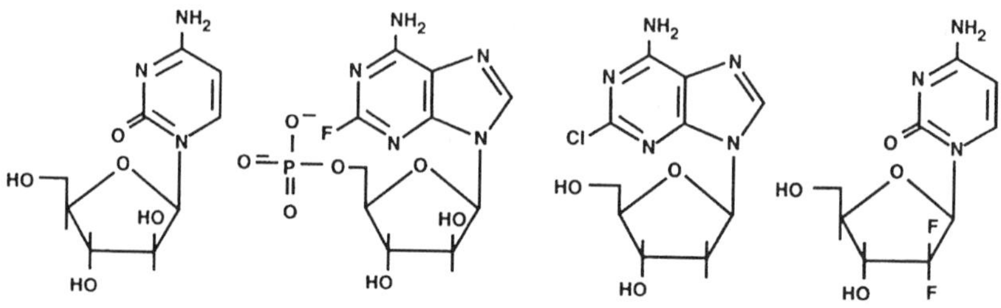

Fig. 1. Structure of clinically used nucleoside analogs.

In 1972, cladribine (2-chloro-2'-deoxyadenosine), a chlorine-substituted adenosine with the natural sugar deoxyribose, was the most active among 20 compounds tested against L-1210 mouse leukemia cells in vivo [7]. The same year, Giblett and colleagues [8] reported that two children who had severe combined immunodeficiency had a lack of ADA, and the conclusion could be drawn that intracellular accumulation of phosphorylated nucleotides is toxic to lymphoid cells. This observation provided a biochemical rationale for cytotoxicity from nucleoside analogs and their potential use as immunosuppressive and anticancer agents [9].

Although effective in preclinical studies, the halogenated purine analogs had long been regarded as being too toxic for clinical use, in part because of problems with the interpretation of toxicity data from mouse studies in relation to dosing in clinical studies. One of the problems was that the activating enzyme dCK is more efficient in humans than in mice; significant severe and unacceptable toxicity occurred when converting drug dosages from mouse studies to phase I studies in humans. Cladribine was developed at the Scripps Institute by Dennis Carson and Ernest Beutler [10–12]. It was considered that the enzymatic profile of lymphoid cells would support activation of nucleosides and result in an accumulation of nucleotides, which would lead to immunosuppression and lymphopenia rather than general myelotoxicity. Petzer and colleagues [13], however, documented that cladribine exerted dose-dependent inhibition of colony formation in various assays, such as colony-formin units erythroid (CFU-E), colony-formin units granulocyte-macrophage (CFU-GM), and burst-formin units erythroid (BFU-E). Because of cladribine's considerable myelotoxicity in humans, it initially was given in high dosages as part of myeloablative conditioning for hematopoietic stem cell transplantation in patients who had refractory leukemia. This usage was not pursued because of severe nephro- and neurotoxicity [12]. In the further development a one-log reduction of the dosage, which led to dosages that are close to those that are being used currently, was given to induce immunosuppression in patients who had rheumatoid arthritis and autoimmune diseases. One such patient was treated with cladribine for autoimmune hemolytic anemia as a consequence of chronic lymphocytic leukemia (CLL), and the observation of rapidly decreasing leukemia cell counts supported the initiation of new phase II protocols in lymphoid malignancies. Single patients who had advanced hairy cell leukemia (HCL) were entered in such a protocol. The first patient who had HCL and was treated with cladribine was unable to receive the scheduled second course because of severe pancytopenia with long-standing fever that eventually was diagnosed as cytomegalovirus reactivation. After recovery it was found that the leukemia had entered a complete and durable remission with no further treatment. Therefore, the second patient who had HCL was observed with no further treatment following the first course of cladribine, and again a complete remission was achieved. The subsequent phase II study with cladribine in HCL confirmed the superior complete remission rate from just one course [14].

Before that, during the 1980s, deoxycoformycin was found to be effective therapy for HCL [15] through a biochemical mechanism similar to that of cladribine, simultaneously with the observation that interferon-α is effective therapy through a different and still not completely identified mode of action [16]. Although deoxycoformycin was less toxic and the responses in HCL were more prompt and durable than with interferons, the latter agents were propagated by the pharmaceutical industries, and became the drugs of choice for almost a decade, until cladribine became widely available. Fludarabine has been studied much less, because the success with cladribine did not allow for studies that delineated the true response rate from fludarabine in HCL; however, early studies suggested reduced efficacy of fludarabine compared with cladribine [17].

MECHANISMS OF ACTION

Nucleoside analogs (see Fig. 1) are prodrugs and have to be activated intracellularly through phosphorylation at the 5'-position to their triphosphate compounds. This phosphorylation is mediated by dCK, and by deoxyguanosine kinase. The phosphorylated analogs are substrates for many enzymes that are involved in DNA synthesis and repair, and are incorporated into DNA in proliferating cells, which leads to cytotoxicity. Nucleoside analogs also are toxic to nondividing cells [18], which is clinically obvious in situations where massive tumor cell reduction and tumor lysis syndrome occur within days of initiating treatment for CLL. This has been interpreted as the result of accumulation of DNA strand breaks because of inhibition of DNA repair, reduction of RNA, and activation of poly(ADP-ribose) polymerase that leads to depletion of NAD^+ and ATP, and, thus, blocks energy-dependent cellular activities.

Cladribine is a strong inhibitor of cholesterol metabolism in vitro [19]. Because cholesterol metabolism is highly active in hairy cells, rich with cell membranes, this might explain why HCL seems to be much more sensitive to the cytotoxic action of cladribine than are other lympho- or myeloproliferative disorders.

More recently, p53-dependent pathways for purine analog toxicity have been identified and proposed to be significant for killing of resting cells through mitochondrial depolarization [20,21]. p53 deletions in CLL were shown to be associated with refractoriness to conventional therapy, including purine analogs, which leads to short survival [22,23]; however, individual patients who have early CLL and p53 aberrations may respond to fludarabine [24]. The compound p53-dependent reactivation and induction of massive apoptosis (PRIMA-1) can restore wild-type conformation and specific DNA binding of mutant p53, and recently was found to be equally cytotoxic in vitro to CLL cells with or without p53 deletions, and also provided synergistic action with fludarabine in p53-deleted CLL cells [25].

An important distinction in cancer therapy is cytotoxicity to clonogenic, self-renewing cancer stem cells, in contrast to the more studied effects on bulk tumor cells. In CLL, a minor proportion of the leukemic cells is proliferating [26,27]; however, clonogenic cells [28] are believed to be predominant in the proliferating centers of the lymph nodes, whereas bulk tumor cells constitute the main tumor cell volume in the peripheral blood and other parts of the lymphoid system. Bulk tumor cells contribute highly to clinical symptoms, but because they are less able to reconstitute relapse their importance for the long-term consequences of the disease is limited. Studies of CLL cell clonogenicity are limited.

CLADRIBINE PHARMACOKINETICS

Initial studies showed that prolonged in vitro exposure was required for cladribine-induced cytotoxicity to leukemia cells. Because insensitive techniques indicated a short initial half-life for cladribine in plasma, with no detectable residual drug 2 hours after infusion in vivo, in early clinical studies the obvious choice was to administer cladribine as a long-term continuous infusion [12]. Continuous infusion for several weeks was tested initially, but was reduced to 7 days; however, for practical reasons schedules that used 2-hour infusions once daily for 5 days also were tested in patients who had CLL or lymphoma, and clinical efficacy also could be documented with intermittent infusions.

Subsequently, high performance liquid chromatography (HPLC) techniques were developed [29] that made it possible to determine the terminal half-life to be 10 hours, which resulted in detectable levels of plasma cladribine 24 hours after infusion of standard doses. More importantly, after infusion intracellular cladribine nucleotides accumulate rapidly to a level that is 2.5 logs higher than the plasma level of the nucleoside (Fig. 2) [30]. Furthermore, the initial half-life of the nucleotides was 13 hours in CLL, and the terminal half-life following the end of the treatment course was 30 hours; intracellular nucleotide levels were recognized 2 weeks after the end of the infusion. Finally, it was shown that the area-under-the-curves—for cladribine in plasma and for cladribine nucleotides in leukemic cells—were similar during and following intermittent infusion as compared with continuous infusion (see Fig. 2) [31]. Therefore, there is no rationale for giving cladribine as a continuous infusion, and the schedule within a treatment course is not likely to influence the therapeutic results, which also was found when various phase II trials were compared.

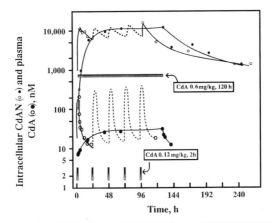

Fig. 2. Concentrations of cladribine (CdA) in plasma and cladribine nucleotides (CdAN) in leukemic cells following intermittent infusion as compared with continuous infusion. There was no difference in AUC between the two modes of administration. Solid lines indicate concentrations from continuous infusion, and dashed lines indicate concentrations from intermittent infusions. (*From* Liliemark J, Juliusson G. Cellular pharmacokinetics of 2-chloro-2′-deoxyadenosine nucleotides: comparison of intermittent and continuous intravenous infusion and subcutaneous and oral administration in leukemia patients. Clin Cancer Res 1995;1(4):387; with permission.)

Studies on the bioavailability indicate that subcutaneous injections provide the same plasma levels as does intravenous (IV) infusion (Fig. 3), with a time to the peak level of about 45 minutes, which corresponds to such a time for IV infusion [31]. In contrast, oral administration leads to partial degradation to chloro-adenine (Fig. 4) [32], which results in a bioavailability of

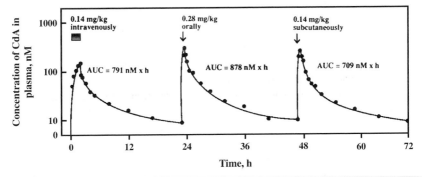

Fig. 3. Plasma concentrations of cladribine (CdA) using three different modes of administration. (*From* Liliemark J, Albertioni F, Hassan M, et al. On the bioavailability of oral and subcutaneous 2-chloro-2′-deoxyadenosine in humans: alternative routes of administration. J Clin Oncol 1992;10(10):1515; with permission.)

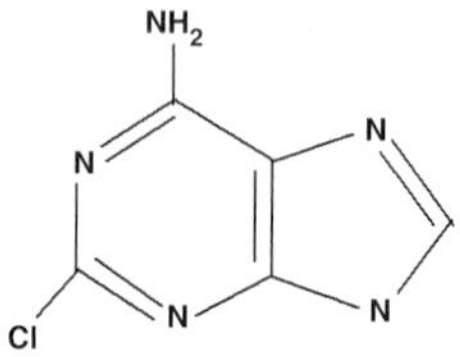

Fig. 4. 2-Chloroadenine.

cladribine of about 40% of the corresponding IV dosage [31,33,34]. With a 2- to 2.5-fold increase of the dosage the plasma level looks similar to that following subcutaneous injections or intravenous infusions for 1 to 2 hours [31]. Subcutaneous injections are tolerated well, and patients do not experience local pain or skin irritation [35]. The initial commercial preparation of cladribine has a concentration of 1 mg/mL, and, thus, large volumes of about 10 mL may be required for standard dose therapy once daily, which has been done regularly without problems. Recently, another preparation with a concentration of 2 mg/mL has been approved and is available in Europe.

Similar to cytosine arabinoside, cladribine penetrates the blood–brain barrier, and spinal fluid levels reach about 25% of the plasma cladribine level [36]. Patients who are treated with the standard dosage of cladribine do not experience neurologic symptoms, such as nausea or vomiting, but it has not been possible to assess if spinal fluid levels are likely to be sufficient for the treatment of central nervous system leukemia. Intraspinal injection of cladribine might be a useful option for treatment of meningeal leukemia, because cladribine is nontoxic to tissues when given subcutaneously or when extravasation occurs, but this has not been evaluated, and therefore, is not recommended.

CLINICAL EXPERIENCE WITH DIFFERENT DRUG ADMINISTRATIONS

Most studies in HCL have been performed using 7-day continuous IV infusion, because this was the routine in early drug development, and the therapeutic success in HCL conserved the schedule; intermittent infusion for 5 days became the established schedule in CLL and lymphoma. The single course of therapy for HCL also made the continuous schedule acceptable, and some institutions were equipped well with infusions pumps and regularly used central catheters, whereas the repeated courses that are required for CLL therapy made this administration form unpractical. Furthermore, central percutaneous catheters increased the risk for phlebitis, which is rare with short-term infusions in peripheral catheters.

The authors and colleagues [35] performed a large study with subcutaneous injection of cladribine for HCL. In this study they chose to mimic the pharmacologic levels that were achieved with the standard 7-day schedule, and, thus, gave 3.4 mg/m^2 once daily for 7 days (total dose 23.8 mg/m^2). The results were positive, with most patients being treated as outpatients and by self-administration. The treatment results, which were confirmed by extensive flow cytometry monitoring [37], showed response rates and response kinetics (Fig. 5) that were comparable to other studies in HCL.

The clinical problem with febrile complications following treatment has been addressed in several ways. First, the addition of granulocyte/macrophage colony-stimulating factor was given in a randomized fashion, but this did not improve complication rates, and did not improve neutrophil counts following

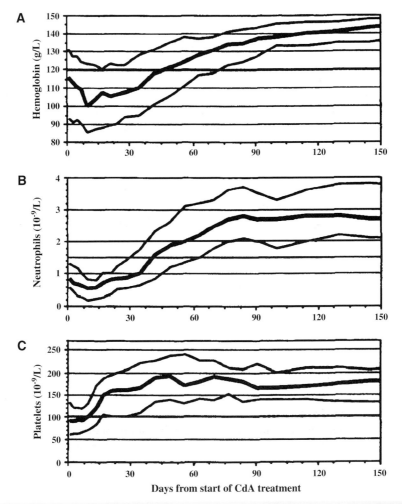

Fig. 5. Recovery from cytopenia following subcutaneous injections of cladribine (CdA) for symptomatic HCL. (*A*) Hemoglobin. (*B*) Neutrophil counts. (*C*) Platelet counts. Lines indicate median and quartile values. (*From* Juliusson G, Heldal D, Hippe E, et al. Subcutaneous injections of 2-chlorodeoxyadenosine for symptomatic hairy cell leukemia. J Clin Oncol 1995;13(4): 990; with permission.)

treatment [38]. Second, the authors and colleagues performed a dose de-escalation study to identify the minimal effective dose. Patients who had early disease with only minor symptoms were given low-dose cladribine. One mg/m^2 daily for 7 days (total dose 7 mg/m^2) did not result in any effect, no decrease in circulating hairy cells, and no change in any blood cell count, including lymphocyte subset counts. These patients received a new course with standard-dose cladribine after 3 months of observation, and then went into complete remission. Thus, the 1 mg/m^2/d dosage was considered to be without effects. A subsequent cohort of patients received 2 mg/m^2 for 7 days (total dose 14 mg/m^2); the response rate and kinetics were the same as for the standard dose, but with less lymphopenia [39]. The dose of 14 mg/m^2 is not much greater than the daily dosage that was given to children who had acute leukemia [40–42], and, therefore, the authors and colleagues evaluated if a single injection would be sufficient treatment for HCL. A single injection of 14 mg/m^2 did result in response and improved blood counts, but the complete remission rate was not as high as with the standard dose; therefore, the single injection schedule was abandoned. The simplified schedule of 5 mg/m^2 daily for 3 days, or 10 mg total daily dosage for 3 days, was shown to be effective and useful in HCL. For other indications and for HCL with a decreased chance for complete remission [35] (eg, patients who have increased lymphocyte counts, variant cell morphology, or aberrant phenotypes), the authors and colleagues usually give five daily dosages of 5 mg/m^2 or up to a 10-mg total dosage per day (total treatment course consists of five vials, each containing 10 mg cladribine). The simplified management of patients who have HCL has decentralized treatment; therefore, the authors and colleagues have not been able to achieve long-term follow-up on patients who receive alternate schedules. The impression is that the response duration is as good as expected, and the response rates from retreatment if required years after initial therapy indicate high new remission rates.

Oral treatment with cladribine is feasible if appropriate dose adjustment is performed, similar to the more recently developed experience with oral fludarabine therapy [43]. The degradation rate and bioavailability of cladribine is predictable, and the interindividual variability is not greater than what has been seen with IV infusions [31]. In CLL and lymphomas where repeated courses are the rule, continuation of therapy could be adjusted according to the initial response and toxicity. By contrast, in HCL response evaluation is performed first after the end of therapy, although an additional course might be given for incomplete response. The authors and colleagues' results from oral cladribine in CLL indicate a similar activity as with parenteral administration [44,45], as expected from the preceding studies on bioavailability and pharmacokinetics. There are no data on oral purine analog treatment of HCL.

In the authors and colleagues' studies oral cladribine was given by drinking a solution of cladribine in saline. This is feasible, but the logistics are impractical; however, oral treatment will improve with the development of a cladribine tablet, which is under evaluation.

SUMMARY

Cladribine is effective therapy for HCL, and there are several ways to achieve the adequate concentrations of the active metabolites in relevant cells, without the need for long-term continuous infusions. This simplifies therapy, although careful control of patients is required during and after treatment in most instances because of the significant activity of the drug on leukemia cells of various types and also on lymphoid cells and normal stem cells.

References

[1] Hitchings GH, Elion GB, Falco EA, et al. Studies on analogs of purines and pyrimidines. Ann N Y Acad Sci 1950;52(8):1318–35.

[2] Elion GB, Hitchings GH, Vanderwerff H. Antagonists of nucleic acid derivatives. VI. Purines. J Biol Chem 1951;192(2):505–18.

[3] Walwick E, Decker C, Roberts W. Cyclization during phosphorylation of uridine and cytidine. A new role to the O2 2' cyclo nucleoside. Proc Chem Soc 1959;53:84.

[4] Dixon RL, Adamson RH. Antitumor activity and pharmacologic disposition of cytosine arabinoside (NSC-63878). Cancer Chemother Rep 1965;48:11–6.

[5] Montgomery JA, Hewson K. Synthesis of potential anticancer agents. XX. 2-Fluoropurines. J Am Chem Soc 1960;82:463–8.

[6] Montgomery JA, Hewson K. Nucleosides of 2-fluoroadenine. J Med Chem 1969;12(3): 498–504.

[7] Christensen LF, Broom AD, Robins MJ, et al. Synthesis and biological activity of selected 2,6-disubstituted-(2-deoxy- -and- -D-erythro-pentofuranosyl) purines. J Med Chem 1972;15(7): 735–9.

[8] Giblett ER, Anderson JE, Cohen F, et al. Adenosine-deaminase deficiency in two patients with severely impaired cellular immunity. Lancet 1972;2(7786):1067–9.

[9] Carson DA, Kaye J, Matsumoto S, et al. Biochemical basis for the enhanced toxicity of deoxyribonucleosides toward malignant human T cell lines. Proc Natl Acad Sci U S A 1979;76(5):2430–3.

[10] Carson DA, Wasson DB, Taetle R, et al. Specific toxicity of 2-chlorodeoxyadenosine toward resting and proliferating human lymphocytes. Blood 1983;62(4):737–43.

[11] Carson DA, Wasson DB, Beutler E. Antileukemic and immunosuppressive activity of 2-chloro-2'-deoxyadenosine. Proc Natl Acad Sci U S A 1984;81(7):2232–6.

[12] Beutler E. Cladribine (2-chlorodeoxyadenosine). Lancet 1992;340(8825):952–6.

[13] Petzer AL, Bilgeri R, Zilian U, et al. Inhibitory effect of 2-chlorodeoxyadenosine on granulocytic, erythroid, and T-lymphocytic colony growth. Blood 1991;78(10):2583–7.

[14] Piro LD, Carrera CJ, Carson DA, et al. Lasting remissions in hairy-cell leukemia induced by a single infusion of 2-chlorodeoxyadenosine. N Engl J Med 1990;322(16): 1117–21.

[15] Spiers AS, Parekh SJ, Bishop MB. Hairy-cell leukemia: induction of complete remission with pentostatin (2'-deoxycoformycin). J Clin Oncol 1984;2(12):1336–42.

[16] Quesada JR, Reuben J, Manning JT, et al. Alpha interferon for induction of remission in hairy-cell leukemia. N Engl J Med 1984;310(1):15–8.

[17] Kantarjian HM, Schachner J, Keating MJ. Fludarabine therapy in hairy cell leukemia. Cancer 1991;67(5):1291–3.

[18] Seto S, Carrera CJ, Kubota M, et al. Mechanism of deoxyadenosine and 2-chlorodeoxyadenosine toxicity to nondividing human lymphocytes. J Clin Invest 1985;75(2): 377–83.

[19] Lechleitner M, Auer B, Zilian U, et al. The immunosuppressive substance 2-chloro-2-deoxyadenosine modulates lipoprotein metabolism in a murine macrophage cell line (P388 cells). Lipids 1994;29(9):627–33.

[20] Pettitt AR, Clarke AR, Cawley JC, et al. Purine analogues kill resting lymphocytes by p53-dependent and -independent mechanisms. Br J Haematol 1999;105(4):986–8.

[21] Pettitt AR. Mechanism of action of purine analogues in chronic lymphocytic leukaemia. Br J Haematol 2003;121(5):692–702.

[22] Fenaux P, Preudhomme C, Lai JL, et al. Mutations of the p53 gene in B-cell chronic lymphocytic leukemia: a report on 39 cases with cytogenetic analysis. Leukemia 1992;6(4):246–50.

[23] Dohner H, Fischer K, Bentz M, et al. p53 gene deletion predicts for poor survival and non-response to therapy with purine analogs in chronic B-cell leukemias. Blood 1995;85(6):1580–9.

[24] Valganon M, Giraldo P, Agirre X, et al. p53 Aberrations do not predict individual response to fludarabine in patients with B-cell chronic lymphocytic leukaemia in advanced stages Rai III/IV. Br J Haematol 2005;129(1):53–9.

[25] Nahi H, Lehmann S, Mollgard L, et al. Effects of PRIMA-1 on chronic lymphocytic leukaemia cells with and without hemizygous p53 deletion. Br J Haematol 2004;127(3):285–91.

[26] Granziero L, Ghia P, Circosta P, et al. Survivin is expressed on CD40 stimulation and interfaces proliferation and apoptosis in B-cell chronic lymphocytic leukemia. Blood 2001;97(9):2777–83.

[27] Bueso-Ramos CE, Ferrajoli A, Medeiros LJ, et al. Aberrant morphology, proliferation, and apoptosis of B-cell chronic lymphocytic leukemia cells. Hematology (Am Soc Hematol Educ Program) 2004;9(4):279–86.

[28] Sala R, Mauro FR, Bellucci R, et al. Evaluation of marrow and blood haemopoietic progenitors in chronic lymphocytic leukaemia before and after chemotherapy. Eur J Haematol 1998;61(1):14–20.

[29] Liliemark J, Pettersson B, Juliusson G. Determination of 2-chloro-2′-deoxyadenosine in human plasma. Biomed Chromatogr 1991;5(6):262–4.

[30] Liliemark J, Juliusson G. Cellular pharmacokinetics of 2-chloro-2′-deoxyadenosine nucleotides: comparison of intermittent and continuous intravenous infusion and subcutaneous and oral administration in leukemia patients. Clin Cancer Res 1995;1(4):385–90.

[31] Liliemark J, Albertioni F, Hassan M, et al. On the bioavailability of oral and subcutaneous 2-chloro-2′-deoxyadenosine in humans: alternative routes of administration. J Clin Oncol 1992;10(10):1514–8.

[32] Lindemalm S, Liliemark J, Juliusson G, et al. Cytotoxicity and pharmacokinetics of cladribine metabolite, 2-chloroadenine in patients with leukemia. Cancer Lett 2004;210(2):171–7.

[33] Saven A, Cheung WK, Smith I, et al. Pharmacokinetic study of oral and bolus intravenous 2-chlorodeoxyadenosine in patients with malignancy. J Clin Oncol 1996;14(3):978–83.

[34] Albertioni F, Juliusson G, Liliemark J. On the bioavailability of 2-chloro-2′-deoxyadenosine (CdA). The influence of food and omeprazole. Eur J Clin Pharmacol 1993;44(6):579–82.

[35] Juliusson G, Heldal D, Hippe E, et al. Subcutaneous injections of 2-chlorodeoxyadenosine for symptomatic hairy cell leukemia. J Clin Oncol 1995;13(4):989–95.

[36] Liliemark J, Juliusson G. On the pharmacokinetics of 2-chloro-2′-deoxyadenosine (CdA) in cerebrospinal fluid (CSF). Blood 1992;80(Suppl 1): 471a.

[37] Juliusson G, Lenkei R, Liliemark J. Flow cytometry of blood and bone marrow cells from patients with hairy cell leukemia: phenotype of hairy cells and lymphocyte subsets after treatment with 2-chlorodeoxyadenosine. Blood 1994;83(12):3672–81.

[38] Juliusson G, Lenkei R, Tjonnfjord G, et al. Neutropenic fever following cladribine therapy for symptomatic hairy-cell leukemia: predictive factors and effects of granulocyte-macrophage colony-stimulating factor. Ann Oncol 1995;6(4):371–5.

[39] Juliusson G, Lenkei R, Tjonnfjord G, et al. Low-dose cladribine for symptomatic hairy cell leukaemia. Br J Haematol 1995;89(3):637–9.

[40] Santana VM, Hurwitz CA, Blakley RL, et al. Complete hematologic remissions induced by 2-chlorodeoxyadenosine in children with newly diagnosed acute myeloid leukemia. Blood 1994;84(4):1237–42.

[41] Krance RA, Hurwitz CA, Head DR, et al. Experience with 2-chlorodeoxyadenosine in previously untreated children with newly diagnosed acute myeloid leukemia and myelodysplastic diseases. J Clin Oncol 2001;19(11):2804–11.

[42] Rubnitz JE, Razzouk BI, Srivastava DK, et al. Phase II trial of cladribine and cytarabine in relapsed or refractory myeloid malignancies. Leuk Res 2004;28(4):349–52.

[43] Boogaerts MA, Van Hoof A, Catovsky D, et al. Activity of oral fludarabine phosphate in previously treated chronic lymphocytic leukemia. J Clin Oncol 2001;19(22): 4252–8.

[44] Juliusson G, Christiansen I, Hansen MM, et al. Oral cladribine as primary therapy for patients with B-cell chronic lymphocytic leukemia. J Clin Oncol 1996;14(7):2160–6.

[45] Karlsson K, Stromberg M, Liliemark J, et al. Oral cladribine for B-cell chronic lymphocytic leukaemia: report of a phase II trial with a 3-d, 3-weekly schedule in untreated and pretreated patients, and a long-term follow-up of 126 previously untreated patients. Br J Haematol 2002;116(3):538–48.

HEMATOLOGY/ONCOLOGY CLINICS
OF NORTH AMERICA

Pentostatin: Impact on Outcome in Hairy Cell Leukemia

Michael R. Grever, MD

Department of Internal Medicine, The Ohio State University, 1654 Upham Drive,
Room 215 Means Hall, Columbus, OH 43210, USA

I n 1958, Bouroncle and colleagues [1] described the clinical and pathologic features of hairy cell leukemia. This rare disease was associated with pancytopenia and profound complications, including infection, that often led to death. Although several other unusual features of this rare entity were of interest, the disease essentially was refractory to therapy until 1984 [2]. Quesada and colleagues [3] reported that α-interferon produced clinical responses, but before this discovery the sole remedy focused upon splenectomy for patients who had hypersplenism and bone marrow failure. The use of standard alkylating agents as chemotherapy was tolerated poorly, and was marginally effective. Therefore, there was enormous enthusiasm for the beneficial effects that were associated with interferon therapy. Interferon administered thrice weekly resulted in a complete remission that approximated 10%, with an overall response rate that approached 80%. Many patients had improvement in their peripheral blood counts, and, thus, were able to deal with infection better.

In 1981, the author and colleagues [4] reported that the administration of pentostatin as a potent inhibitor of adenosine deaminase produced clinical responses in patients who had advanced chronic lymphoid leukemias. In contrast, earlier trials that used much higher dosages of this agent for treating patients who had acute leukemia were unsuccessful. Excessive toxicity, characterized by immunosuppression and nephrotoxicity, was encountered with high dosages of pentostatin. In patients who had chronic forms of lymphoid leukemia, the specific activity of the target enzyme, adenosine deaminase, in the leukemic cells was low in comparison to that found in acute leukemia [4,5]. Spiers and colleagues [6] reported that using this low-dose administration of pentostatin in a limited number of patients who had hairy cell leukemia resulted in complete hematologic remission. Furthermore, Kraut and colleagues [7] confirmed that 9 of 10 patients who had hairy cell leukemia achieved a complete hematologic remission when this agent was administered at 4 mg/m^2 by intravenous bolus once every 14 days. This low-dose regimen delivered in an out-patient setting was effective and was tolerated extremely

E-mail address: michael.grever@osumc.edu

0889-8588/06/$ – see front matter
doi:10.1016/j.hoc.2006.06.001

well. In fact, the administration of pentostatin was associated with marked patient improvement in a larger study without excessive risk for infection [8].

Additional investigators showed that the achievement of a complete remission exceeded 75%; however, some reports did not confirm this level of complete remission [9–11]. The author and colleagues [11] showed that patients who have older age, enlarged spleens, and severe anemia were statistically less likely to achieve a complete remission. These clinical differences between patient populations and the likelihood that some case reports included patients who had received previous therapy may explain some of the disparate results. Nevertheless, the overwhelming number of separate clinical experiences showed that the complete remissions were achievable and durable. In general, patients who were infected actively at the time of initiating therapy with pentostatin did as well as those who were not infected [11]. Habermann and colleagues [12], however, recommended that initial therapy with interferon followed by pentostatin was an alternative strategy for patients who have active infection at the time of initial therapy.

The lowest dosage of pentostatin that is capable of inducing a complete remission was never defined carefully. The studies that used less intensive dosages were associated with the higher complete remission rates (Table 1).

A subset of patients that has hairy cell leukemia presents with a severely hypocellular marrow that may be difficult to distinguish from aplastic anemia [13]. In patients who present with a severely hypocellular bone marrow, a complete remission with pentostatin is achievable [14]. These patients may be unusually susceptible to the myelosuppressive effects of cytotoxic chemotherapy. To avoid a prolonged period of worsening myelosuppression, patients with a hypocellular presentation have been treated with initial dosages of pentostatin that are as low as 2 mg/m^2 intravenously every 2 to 3 weeks [8]. As the peripheral blood counts begin to improve, the dosages of pentostatin can be increased gradually to the standard dosage of 4 mg/m^2 intravenously every 2 to 4 weeks.

In general, patients who have achieved the most durable remissions have been treated with pentostatin for periods of 4 to 12 months on an alternate

Table 1
Complete remissions with pentostatin in hairy cell leukemia

Study	N	Complete remission rate (%)	Dosage & schedule
Kraut et al [8]	23	87	2–4 mg/m^2 IV q 14 d
Johnston et al [9]	28	89	4 mg/m^2 IV weekly × 3 q 8 wk
Else et al [20]	185	81	4 mg/m^2 IV weekly ×4, then q 2 wk (first cohort). Second cohort received 4 mg/m^2 IV q 2 wk.
Grever et al [11]	154	76	2–4 mg/m^2 IV q 2 wk

Abbreviations: IV, intravenously; q, every.

week schedule in the out-patient setting [8,11]. For patients with a good performance status and a cellular bone marrow, the usual dosage of pentostatin (4 mg/m^2) is given as an intravenous bolus every 2 weeks until maximal response has occurred, including achievement of a complete remission on bone marrow examination by light microscopy. Although patients may have experienced complete recovery of their peripheral blood counts, the bone marrow aspirate and biopsy frequently show some residual hairy cell leukemia by immunohistochemical staining [15]. Therefore, most of the reported successful studies have discontinued therapy after the disappearance of histologic evidence of hairy cell leukemia in the bone marrow and regression of splenomegaly by physical examination. Recent studies have used the extent of minimal residual disease to predict relapse [16]. Consequently, future trials may focus on strategies to eliminate the minimal residual disease by adding other agents (eg, Rituxan) or by combining agents within the context of new clinical trials. In the setting of routine practice, most hematologists administer the agent until a complete remission has been achieved or until 6 to 12 months of therapy have been delivered.

Over the past few years, long-term follow-up has shown that pentostatin has changed the natural history of this form of chronic leukemia (Table 2) [11,17–20]. Many patients have remained in remission at 5 years and at 10 years. In patients who relapsed (and required retreatment), there is a variable reported

Table 2
Long-term outcome with pentostatin in hairy cell leukemia

Study	N	Outcome data
Else et al [20]	185	Patient median follow-up 10.8 years. Overall survival at 10 years is 96% with 5-year relapse rate is 24% and 10-year relapse rate is 42%; estimated median disease-free survival is 15 years.
Flinn et al [26]	173	Patient median follow-up 9.3 years. 5-year relapse free survival is 85%, and 10-year relapse-free survival is 67%. Relapse rate in those with a complete remission is 18%.
Johnston et al [19]	28	Patient median follow-up 9.8 years. Relapse-free survival at 5 years is 80%; relapse-free survival at 10 years is 76%.
Ribeiro et al [18]	50	Many patients were treated previously with interferon, splenectomy, or other agents. Overall survival after pentostatin is 86% at 38 months of follow-up. The previously untreated patients who responded had not progressed at 21 months of follow-up.

second complete remission rate of 44% to 75% [11,17]. Compared with the previous expected survival of 4 to 4.5 years for patients who have hairy cell leukemia before the introduction of the purine nucleoside analogs, the average survival is now close to a normal age-matched patient population [11]. Therefore, the extensive work in purine nucleoside drug development clearly has changed the natural history of this previously fatal disease.

In 1990, cladribine, another purine nucleoside analog, showed remarkable ability to induce a complete remission in previously untreated patients who had hairy cell leukemia [21]. There have been numerous subsequent studies with this agent that documented equally spectacular results in producing high rates of complete and durable remissions in this disease [22–25]. Therefore, cladribine and pentostatin produce comparable high complete remission rates, yet there is microscopic residual leukemia in many of these patients (eg, examined by specialized immunohistochemical stains) [15,16]. Because the rate of relapse using either agent is comparable, and there is no plateau in the disease-free survival curves, neither drug is capable of curing these patients.

RELAPSE IN PATIENTS WHO HAVE HAIRY CELL LEUKEMIA

The rates for relapse vary between trials, but, in general, are in agreement. Flinn and colleagues [26] reported on 241 patients who were treated with pentostatin for hairy cell leukemia. With a median follow-up of 9.3 years, including data on 173 patients who had achieved a confirmed complete remission, the relapse rate was 18%. The projected 5-year relapse-free survival was 85%, and the 10-year projected relapse-free survival was 67%. Else and colleagues [20] reported on 185 patients who were treated with pentostatin with a median follow-up from diagnosis of 12.5 years. In that report, the relapse rate at 5 years for patients who achieved a complete remission with pentostatin was 24%, whereas the 10 year-rate was 42%.

Patients who achieve complete remission with pentostatin as first-line therapy have a prolonged disease-free survival (DFS) compared with those who have a partial remission. Furthermore, there is a correlation with the extent of minimal residual disease demonstrated by immunohistochemical staining of the bone marrow biopsy with DBA.44 and subsequent relapse. Flow cytometric techniques also can be used to search for circulating minimal residual disease. Although many patients can function extremely well in the face of minimal residual disease, there has been no consistent approach to patients with this finding. Many patients simply are followed until there is clear demonstration of progressive disease or deterioration in the patient's peripheral blood counts that necessitates retreatment. It is important to avoid delaying retreatment until the peripheral blood counts have decreased to low values.

Patients who have had prolonged DFS following initial therapy have a high chance of responding to retreatment with pentostatin. Repeat administration of pentostatin achieved a second complete remission in approximately 60% of patients in Else and colleagues' [20] experience; however, each subsequent relapse is expected to have a progressively shorter DFS and a lower overall achievement of a complete remission. In general, there is little systematic data regarding the response of patients to other purine nucleosides following failure of pentostatin. Patients have been reported to respond to pentostatin or cladribine following failure to the initial respective agent [24,25]. Furthermore, patients who fail a purine nucleoside analog have responded to Rituxan [27]. In limited numbers of patients, Rituxan also has been used to eradicate minimal residual disease. Finally, patients who fail to respond to a purine nucleoside analog or interferon have responded to immunotoxin conjugates that are directed at CD22 or CD25 [27]. The intriguing concept that using a biologic agent to convert minimal residual disease into a complete remission requires further systematic evaluation in the context of a clinical trial.

Finally, patients who have failed to respond to a purine nucleoside analog or to a biologic agent may derive some benefit from a trial of interferon [27,28]. The potential benefit to interferon is limited, but it may be useful for patients who have not responded to the purine nucleoside analogs. Furthermore, there may be a role for the use of interferon initially in patients who require treatment but have an active infection.

Splenectomy also may offer a temporizing benefit for patients who have pancytopenia and an enlarged spleen [2,27]. There are a few important remaining indications for considering splenectomy in the current management of hairy cell leukemia. In patients who have severe thrombocytopenia and active bleeding, splenectomy still may be the treatment of choice for patients who have an enlarged spleen. The response of the platelets to purine nucleoside analogs may take a few weeks, and severely thrombocytopenic patients with a serious potential for bleeding may not respond in sufficient time for safety. Therefore, in patients with poor response to standard agents, it is important to reconsider the accuracy of the diagnosis and consider alternative therapy.

It is important to confirm the diagnosis of hairy cell leukemia in patients who have failed to respond to the usual agents. In patients who have the variant of hairy cell leukemia, the response to purine nucleoside analogs is not as impressive or durable compared with the standard form of the disease.

IMMUNOSUPPRESSIVE EFFECTS OF PENTOSTATIN IN PATIENTS WHO HAVE HAIRY CELL LEUKEMIA

Pentostatin is immunosuppressive, and patients who have hairy cell leukemia also have an underlying propensity to infection as a result of impaired immune effector cell function [29,30]. Consequently, patients who are being treated with a purine nucleoside analog must be followed carefully for opportunistic infection. The contribution of the purine nucleoside analogs to decreasing the T cell numbers and impairing their function may contribute to the increased risk for infection. Many of the patients who have been treated successfully with pentostatin are treated simultaneously with prophylaxis for *Pneumocystis carinii* and viral diseases. The required duration of this prophylaxis is determined empirically based upon observations that defects in the residual T-cell compartments of these patients persist for up to a year. In several large clinical trials with several hundreds of patients, it is encouraging that there have been few long-term consequences of serious infection [26,30,31].

Patients who have hairy cell leukemia are prone to develop granulocytopenia immediately following the initial therapy with pentostatin or cladribine. Approximately 14% of patients who were treated with pentostatin developed grade 4 granulocytopenia, and this may be lessened by using lower initial doses of the drug or potentially by using granulocyte colony-stimulating factor (G-CSF) [32]. In patients who have a history of vasculitis, some investigators have advised that G-CSF may exacerbate this complication of the underlying disease [33].

Infection is one of the major concerns with hairy cell leukemia and its treatment. The frequency of febrile neutropenia that required initiation of a systemic antibiotic following pentostatin was 27% in one large trial, and this seems to be less than that reported in other studies that used cladribine to treat the leukemia (ie, 37%–58%) [21,24,25]. As patients begin to respond to pentostatin, the dosages may be adjusted upward toward the standard dosage of 4 mg/m^2 delivered intravenously every 2 to 3 weeks. Patients may tolerate this gradual increase in dosage following improvement in their pretreatment granulocyte and platelet counts. Most of the therapy may be delivered in the out-patient clinic, and periods of drug-induced myelosuppression may be avoided by judiciously adjusting the dosage and schedule of drug administration. A delay of 1 or 2 weeks may result in continued improvement in the peripheral blood counts while the patient improves with respect to symptoms from the disease [5,8].

Long-term follow-up on studies that used pentostatin to treat hairy cell leukemia have not demonstrated an increased risk for the development of a second malignancy [17–20,26]. Cheson and colleagues [34] conducted an analysis of the long-term risks associated with treatment in several trials, and specifically concluded that there was no increase in second malignancies following the use of pentostatin. Although there may have been a slight increase in the risk for a second malignancy associated with other purine analogs, this has not been the case with pentostatin in patients who were followed for 10 to 12 years after therapy. The quality and the quantity of life for patients who have hairy cell leukemia have been improved markedly with the use of pentostatin as first-line therapy for this disease.

PRACTICAL CONSIDERATIONS: PENTOSTATIN FOR HAIRY CELL LEUKEMIA

The results of multiple trials have defined the use of a purine nucleoside analog as the therapy of choice for patients who have hairy cell leukemia. Although the overall survival of patients has been improved markedly with a single agent, there is increasing realization that multiple agents may result in a "more complete remission." For example, the use of Rituxan to eradicate minimal residual disease will need to be explored carefully in the future. Pentostatin is a reasonable choice as front-line therapy. Numerous reports including short- and long-term analysis have confirmed that the results with pentostatin are just as impressive as those observed with cladribine. In fact, no difference exists between these agents with respect to the response or survival [27].

Although the initial use of cladribine offers convenience of one course, there seems to be a higher reported frequency of a requirement for systemic antibiotics compared with a large trial using pentostatin [5]. Patients who were treated with cladribine also were excluded intentionally from participation in the face of an ongoing active infection [21–25]. In contrast, a large clinical trial that compared the safety and efficacy of treatment with pentostatin or interferon did not exclude patients who had infection [5]. In the management of this disease, patients inevitably will be encountered who present for treatment with active infection. Although the preferred approach is to treat the infection successfully before treating the leukemia, this may not be feasible. Patients who were randomized to receive pentostatin had a higher frequency of myelosuppression and infection compared with those who were treated with interferon, but there was no statistical difference in the achievement of a complete remission in the presence of infection between the treatment arms [5]. In considering therapeutic strategies, Habermann and colleagues [12] recommended that initial therapy with interferon followed by pentostatin after improvement in the infection is a reasonable approach. Studies by Kraut and colleagues [8] confirmed that low dosages of pentostatin are effective in inducing a high degree of complete remission (ie, 87%) with an acceptable complication rate with respect to infection.

Pentostatin can be delivered as a rapid intravenous injection in the out-patient setting at a dosage of 4 mg/m^2 every 2 weeks. For patients with an initial Eastern Cooperative Oncology Group (ECOG) performance status of 3, the initial dosage of pentostatin is 2 mg/m^2; subsequent dosages are increased as discussed above if no adverse side effects are observed. Patients are evaluated carefully for the status of renal function at each treatment, because this agent is cleared through a renal route [5]. Therefore, patients who have impaired renal function must have a dosage reduction or be excluded from receiving the purine nucleoside. The serum creatinine should be checked before each dosage of the drug. Hydration with approximately 1.5 L of intravenous fluid is administered while the serum creatinine is being checked. If an increase in serum creatinine is observed that is greater than 20% greater than the baseline, the drug is not administered until renal function is improved to baseline or a 24-hour creatinine clearance confirms that the clearance is greater than 50 mL/min.

When a complete remission has been achieved as confirmed by a bone marrow biopsy, the drug is stopped or two additional doses of pentostatin have been administered (14 days apart). There are no data to support the administration of maintenance drug. Patients are followed closely with peripheral blood counts, and retreatment has been started for patients who have a confirmed relapse. In patients with extensive treatment before achieving a complete remission, prophylaxis for opportunistic infection has been used. The guidelines for the adjunctive use of prophylaxis or the use of G-CSF are under development. If additional immunosuppression is planned (eg, prednisone) following a purine nucleoside analog, it seems that prophylaxis is needed. The duration of administration of these agents and the optimal regimen for infection prevention have not been defined. Close follow-up should be used until there is evidence of recovery of T cells and normal peripheral blood counts.

SUMMARY

Major advances in the management of patients who have hairy cell leukemia have been made following the use of purine nucleoside analogs. Pentostatin and cladribine are equally effective, and have impressive long-term effectiveness. Although the degree of myelosuppression may be less with the use of pentostatin, this may reflect differences in the schedule and dose of drug administration between these agents. The gradual, but relentless, improvement in the peripheral blood counts enables out-patient management with pentostatin in most patients. Cladribine affords the convenience of a single course of administration. A direct comparative study with these two agents is unlikely to yield dramatic differences in improvement. In contrast, future studies to determine the optimal management of patients who have minimal residual disease following the administration of either agent is warranted in the context of a clinical trial. Patients do relapse, and the overall survival curves have not reached a plateau, which indicates that cure has not been secured. The satisfaction of having improved the outcome for patients who have this previously untreatable leukemia should not give way to complacency for further improvement in the management of this disease. Future studies should be directed to optimizing the therapy for minimal residual disease as well as clearer definition of supportive care.

References

[1] Bouroncle BA, Wiseman B, Doan CA. Leukemic reticuloendotheliosis. Blood 1958;13: 609–30.
[2] Zakarija A, Peterson LC, Tallman MS. Splenectomy and treatments of historical interest. Best Pract Res Clin Haematol 2003;16(1):57–69.
[3] Quesada JR, Reuben J, Manning JT, et al. Alpha interferon for induction of remission in hairy-cell leukemia. N Engl J Med 1984;310(1):15–8.
[4] Grever MR, Siaw MF, Jacob WF, et al. The biochemical and clinical consequences of 2′-deoxycoformycin in refractory lymphoproliferative malignancy. Blood 1981;57(3):406–17.
[5] Grever MR, Leiby JM, Kraut EH, et al. Low dose deoxycoformycin in lymphoid malignancy. J Clin Oncol 1985;3(9):1196–201.
[6] Spiers ASD, Parekh SJ, Bishop MB. Hairy cell leukemia: induction of complete remission with pentostatin (2′deoxycoformycin). J Clin Oncol 1984;2:1336–42.
[7] Kraut EH, Bouroncle BA, Grever MR. Low-dose deoxycoformycin in the treatment of hairy cell leukemia. Blood 1986;68(5):1119–22.
[8] Kraut EH, Bouroncle BA, Grever MR. Pentostatin in the treatment of advanced hairy cell leukemia. J Clin Oncol 1989;7(2):168–72.
[9] Johnston JB, Eisenhauer E, Corbett WE, et al. Efficacy of 2′deoxycoformycin in hairy-cell leukemia: a study of the National Cancer Institute of Canada Clinical Trials Group. J Natl Cancer Inst 1988;80(10):765–9.
[10] Spiers AS, Moore D, Cassileth PA, et al. Remissions in hairy-cell leukemia with pentostatin (2′-deoxycoformycin). N Engl J Med 1987;316(14):825–30.

[11] Grever MR, Kopecky K, Head D, et al. Randomized comparison of pentostatin versus inter-feron alpha-2a in previously untreated patients with hairy cell leukemia: an intergroup study. J Clin Oncol 1995;13(4):974–82.

[12] Habermann TM, Andersen JW, Cassileth PA, et al. Sequential administration of recombinant interferon alpha and deoxycoformycin in the treatment of hairy cell leukemia. Br J Haematol 1992;80(4):466–71.

[13] Lee WM, Beckstead JH. Hairy cell leukemia with bone marrow hypoplasia. Cancer 1982;50(10):2207–10.

[14] Ng JP, Nolan B, Chan-Lam D, et al. Successful treatment of aplastic variant of hairy cell leukemia with deoxycoformycin. Hematology (Am Soc Hematol Educ Program) 2002;7(4):259–62.

[15] Tallman MS, Hakiman D, Kopecky KJ, et al. Minimal residual disease in patients with hairy cell leukemia in complete remission treated with 2-chlorodeoxyadenosine or 2-deoxycofor-mycin and prediction of early relapse. Clin Cancer Res 1999;5(7):1665–70.

[16] Mhawech-Fauceglia P, Oberholzer M, Aschenafi S, et al. Potential predictive patterns of minimal residual disease detected by immunohistochemistry on bone marrow biopsy spec-imens during a long-term follow-up in patients treated with cladribine for hairy cell leukemia. Arch Pathol Lab Med 2006;130:374–7.

[17] Kraut EH, Bouroncle BA, Grever MR. Long term follow-up of patients with hairy cell leukemia following treatment with 2'-deoxycoformycin. Blood 1994;84(12):4061–3.

[18] Ribeiro P, Bouaffia F, Peaud PY, et al. Long term outcome of patients with hairy cell leukemia treated with pentostatin. Cancer 1999;85(1):65–71.

[19] Johnston JB, Eisenhauer E, Wainman N, et al. Long term outcome following treatment of hairy cell leukemia with pentostatin (Nipent): a National Cancer Institute of Canada study. Semin Oncol 2000;27 (2)(Suppl 5):32–6.

[20] Else M, Ruchlemer R, Osuji N, et al. Long remissions in hairy cell leukemia with purine analogs: a report of 219 patients with a median follow-up of 12.5 years. Cancer 2005; 104(11):2442–8.

[21] Piro LD, Carrera CJ, Carson DA, et al. Lasting remissions in hairy cell leukemia induced by a single infusion of 2-chlorodeoxyadenosine. N Engl J Med 1990;322(16):1117–21.

[22] Saven A, Burian C, Koziol JA, et al. Long-term followup of patients with hairy cell leukemia after cladribine therapy. Blood 1998;92(6):1918–26.

[23] Saven A, Burian C, Adusumaalli J, et al. Filgrastim for cladribine-induced neutropenic fever in patients with hairy cell leukemia. Blood 1999;93(8):2471–7.

[24] Estey E, Kurzrock R, Kantarjian HM, et al. Treatment of hairy cell leukemia with 2-chloro-deoxyadenosine. Blood 1992;79:882–7.

[25] Juliusson G, Liliemark J. Rapid Recovery from cytopenia in hairy cell leukemia after treat-ment with 2-chloro-2'-deoxyadenosine (CdA): relation to opportunistic infection. Blood 1992;79(4):888–94.

[26] Flinn IW, Kopecky KJ, Foucar MK, et al. Long-term follow-up of remission duration, mortality, and second malignancies in hairy cell leukemia patients treated with pentostatin. Blood 2000;96(9):2981–6.

[27] Mey U, Strehl J, Gorschluter M, et al. Advances in the treatment of hairy cell leukemia. Lancet Oncol 2003;4(2):86–94.

[28] Ahmed S, Rai KR. Interferon in the treatment of hairy cell leukemia. Best Pract Res Clin Hae-matol 2003;16(1):69–81.

[29] Kraut EH, Neff JC, Bouroncle BA, et al. Immunosuppressive effects of pentostatin. J Clin Oncol 1990;8(5):848–55.

[30] Kraut EH. Clinical manifestations and infectious complications of hairy cell leukemia. Best Pract Res Clin Haematol 2003;16(1):33–40.

[31] Ho AD, Mannel DN, Wulf G, et al. Long-term effects of 2'-deoxycoformycin on cytokine production in patients with hairy cell leukemia. Leukemia 1990;4(8):584–9.

[32] Glaspy JA, Souza L, Scates S, et al. Treatment of hairy cell leukemia with granulocyte colony-stimulating factor and recombinant consensus interferon or recombinant interferon-alpha-2b. J Immunother 1992;11(3):198–208.
[33] Saven A, Piro LD. Treatment of hairy cell leukemia. Blood 1992;79(5):1111–20.
[34] Cheson BD, Vena DA, Barrett J, et al. Second malignancies as a consequence of nucleoside analog therapy for chronic lymphoid leukemias. J Clin Oncol 1999;17(8):2454–60.

HEMATOLOGY/ONCOLOGY CLINICS
OF NORTH AMERICA

Cladribine in Hairy Cell Leukemia

Rajesh Belani, MD[a], Alan Saven, MD[a,b,*]

[a]Division of Hematology/Oncology, M/S 217, Scripps Clinic, 10666 North Torrey Pines Road, La Jolla, CA 92037, USA
[b]Ida M. and Cecil H. Green Cancer Center, 10666 North Torrey Pines Road, La Jolla, CA 92037, USA

Hairy cell leukemia (HCL) is a rare chronic B-cell lymphoid malignancy with a greater incidence in elderly men. Patients typically present with splenomegaly, pancytopenia, and recurrent infections. Lymphocytes with characteristic projections are found in the peripheral blood, and they have a characteristic pattern of infiltration in the bone marrow.

Most patients who have HCL require treatment at presentation or some time in their disease course. Usual indications for treatment include platelet counts less than 100×10^9/L, hemoglobin less than 8 to 10 g/dL, absolute neutrophil count (ANC) less than 0.5×10^9/L—or much less commonly—symptomatic splenomegaly or painful lymphadenopathy, recurrent or serious infections, vasculitis, and bony involvement. A variety of agents is effective in the treatment of HCL. Historically, interferon-α and splenectomy were the treatments of choice; however, neither is curative. Splenectomy results in temporary improvement of cytopenias with more than half of the patients requiring systemic treatment within 1 year [1,2].

The most active agents in HCL are the purine analogs. Three purine nucleoside analogs are commercially available in the United States: fludarabine, pentostatin (2'-deoxycoformycin), and cladribine (2-chlorodeoxyadenosine, 2-CdA). Only pentostatin and cladribine have been evaluated extensively in HCL.

In 1972 Giblett and colleagues [3] made the important discovery of adenosine deaminase (ADA) deficiency in children who had severe combined immunodeficiency syndrome. Cohen and colleagues [4] showed that the intracellular accumulation of purine nucleotides was toxic to lymphocytes. Lymphocytes possess high levels of deoxycytidine kinase and low levels of 5'-nucleotidase [5]. ADA is the major pathway for deoxypurine nucleoside's degradation in lymphocytes. Carson and colleagues [5] evaluated several purine nucleoside analogs that were resistant to ADA. Cladribine was one of the agents that was screened and was selected because of its potent in vitro activity against

*Corresponding author. E-mail address: saven.alan@scrippshealth.org (A. Saven).

0889-8588/06/$ – see front matter
doi:10.1016/j.hoc.2006.06.008

lymphocytes [6]. The application of cladribine to the treatment of HCL is reviewed.

SYNTHESIS AND MECHANISM OF ACTION

The efficacy of cladribine likely is related to the specific activation pathways for purine metabolism in lymphocytes. ADA is extremely important for lymphocyte purine metabolism by regulating intracellular levels of adenosine by deamination of adenosine to inosine, and of 2'-deoxyadenosine to 2'-deoxyinosine. Carson and colleagues [7] synthesized several purine analogs that were resistant to degradation by ADA. Cladribine, or 2-chlorodeoxyadenosine was one of the compounds that was synthesized by substituting the hydrogen atom with a chlorine atom at the 2-position of the carbon ring (Fig. 1). These compounds retained their substrate specificity for deoxycytidine kinase. Cladribine was chosen because of its potency and lymphocyte specificity. In vitro, it is more toxic to T lymphoblastoid cell lines than B cells. It induces a lymphopenic state similar to that observed in ADA deficiency.

Cladribine enters the cell by way of a purine nucleotide transporter and is phosphorylated by deoxycytidine kinase to 2-chlorodeoxyadenosine 5'-triphosphate (2-CdATP) (Fig. 2). 2-CdATP is the putative active metabolite of cladribine that is incorporated into DNA and produces strand breaks. Induction of these strand breaks ultimately leads to cell death [6]. 2-CdATP also inhibits ribonucleotide reductase, which reduces the intracellular concentration of deoxynucleotides and inhibits DNA synthesis [8].

A special feature of cladribine is its cytotoxicity to nondividing lymphoid cells. This aspect makes it especially active against indolent lymphoid malignancies. Leoni and colleagues [9] suggested that 2-CdATP may interact directly with cytochrome c and caspase-9, and, thereby, initiate the proteolytic cascade that culminates in apoptosis. Genini and colleagues [10] showed that 2-CdATP activates caspase-9 in cell free extracts. Hairy cells have high deoxycytidine kinase, and low 5'nucleotidase activity. This results in 2-CdATP intracellular

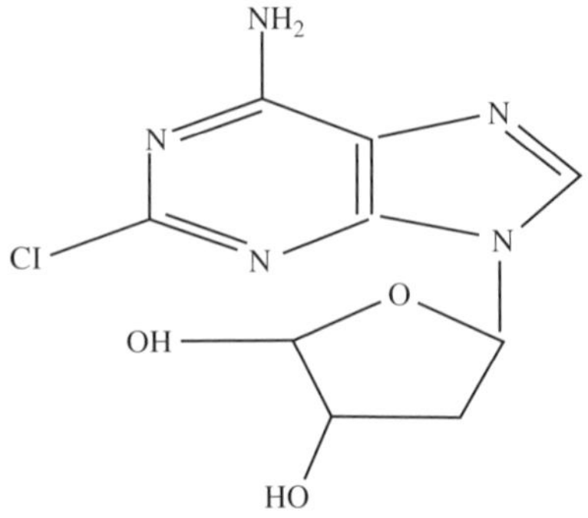

Fig. 1. Structure of cladribine. The hydrogen atom at the 2-position of the purine ring has been substituted with a chloride atom.

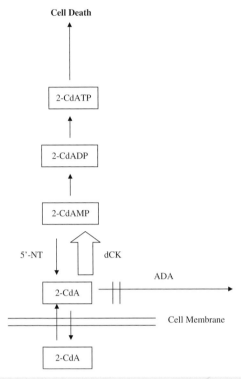

Fig. 2. Mechanism of action of cladribine. Accumulation of 2-CdATP leads to apoptosis. 2-CdADP, 2-chlorodeoxyadenosine 5'-biphosphate; 2-CdAMP, 2-chlorodeoxyadenosine 5'-triphosphate; 5'NT, 5' nucleotidase; dCK, deoxycytidine kinase.

accumulation, which causes nicotinamide adenine dinucleotide (NAD) depletion by activation of a poly-ADP ribose synthetase. NAD is responsible for the metabolism of oxygen radicals. NAD depletion ultimately results in cell death [11].

Monocytes also are vulnerable to cladribine exposure [12,13]. It was suggested that monocytes produce cytokines that support hairy cell survival. Therefore, cladribine may affect hairy cell survival indirectly by disrupting the supporting monocyte network.

Christensen and colleagues [14] first synthesized cladribine by the direct fusion alkylation of 2,6-dichloropurine. Scripps investigators synthesized cladribine from thymidine and 2-chloroadenine using a transdeoxyriboxylase that was derived from *Lactobacillus helveticus* [7]. Cladribine is now manufactured commercially nonenzymatically by using a sodium salt glycosylation procedure.

PHARMACOLOGY AND DOSING SCHEMAS

Cladribine undergoes renal catabolism through its organic cation carrier system. A two-compartment model best defines its elimination kinetics; α and β half-lives are 35 minutes and 6.7 hours, respectively [15]. The 7-day continuous administration of 0.1 mg/kg/d achieves a steady state concentration of 20 to 30 nM. This concentration exceeds the observed in vitro IC_{50} against lymphoid neoplasms [16]. Cladribine is unstable at low pH and is degraded rapidly by bacterial phosphorylases [17]. In HCL, cladribine is administered as a continuous 7-day infusion dissolved in 0.9% sodium chloride at a dosage of 0.085 to 0.1 mg/kg/d.

Alternative methods of cladribine administration have been investigated (Table 1). The safety and tolerability of 0.14 mg/kg/d by a 2-hour bolus infusion for 5 days was compared with 0.1 mg/kg/d continuous infusion for 7 days—same total dose per course. Ninety patients who had relapsed chronic lymphocytic leukemia were enrolled in this study. Response rates and toxicities were identical in the two arms [18]. Juliusson and colleagues [19] treated 73 patients with cladribine at 0.085 mg/kg/d by subcutaneous injection for 7 days. The complete response rate was 81%, with another 15% of patients achieving partial responses. Toxicities were similar to the continuous intravenous (IV) infusion schedule. The bioavailability of subcutaneously administered cladribine compared with the IV infusion is 100%. Lauria and colleagues [20] administered six weekly infusions of cladribine at a dosage of 0.15 mg/kg/wk, each over 2 hours. Twenty-five patients who had HCL were so treated, and the toxicities were comparable to the continuous infusion regimens. The overall response rate was 100%, with 76% achieving complete responses.

Scripps Clinic investigators studied the oral administration of cladribine. Cladribine was administered at a dosage of 0.28 mg/kg orally daily for five consecutive days. Patients swished the solution before swallowing, and omeprazole, 20 mg, was administered before to decrease the gastric acid levels. Four weeks later the patients received cladribine, 0.14 mg/kg/d, by a two-hour IV infusion for five consecutive days. The oral bioavailability of cladribine was 37% to 55%. Cladribine can be administered safely orally at twice the IV dosage to achieve equivalent serum concentrations [21].

These alternative methods of cladribine delivery have not been tested in large numbers of patients who have HCL. Therefore, the authors recommend dosing cladribine at 0.1 mg/kg/d by continuous IV infusion for 7 days as therapy for patients who have HCL. These alternate IV-dosing schedules may be appropriate for selected patients.

Table 1
Alternate dosing schedules for cladribine in hairy cell leukemia

Investigators	Cladribine dosage and route	N	CR (%)	PR (%)
Juliusson et al [19]	0.085 mg/kg/d SQ × 7 days	73	81	15
Lauria et al [20]	0.15 mg/kg/wk IV × 6 weeks	25	76	24

Abbreviations: CR, complete remission; IV, intravenously; PR, partial remission; SQ, subcutaneously.

PRECLINICAL ACTIVITY

B-cell and T-cell malignant lymphoid cell lines and resting peripheral blood lymphocytes are sensitive to cladribine [7,8]. Prolonged in vitro exposure of resting peripheral blood lymphocytes resulted in greater cell death than did brief incubations [16]. This observation provided the rationale for prolonged IV infusions in the initial clinical studies. Cladribine has in vivo antileukemic activity against the L1210 mouse leukemia model.

In preclinical studies, cladribine at a single dosage of 150 mg/kg/d was lethal to 50% of mice. A daily dosage of 100 mg/d was lethal to 50% of mice [22]. In primate studies cladribine at a dosage of 1 mg/kg/d caused severe diarrhea and granulocytopenia [16].

CLINICAL ACTIVITY IN HAIRY CELL LEUKEMIA

Cladribine was tested first in clinical trials that were performed at Scripps Clinic in La Jolla, California. Carrera and colleagues [23] reported the profound activity of cladribine in a patient who had HCL. Two patients who had HCL and failed splenectomy were treated with a single infusion of cladribine; both achieved a complete remission. Later, the same group reported on 12 patients who had HCL who were treated with a single infusion of cladribine; 11 achieved a complete remission [24]. Cladribine was administered as a continuous 7-day infusion at 0.085 mg/kg/d.

Scripps Clinic investigators have reported the largest series of HCL patients treated with cladribine. Saven and colleagues [25] reported their experience with 358 patients who were treated with cladribine; 179 were untreated previously, 95 had undergone splenectomy, 132 had received interferon-α, and 8 had been treated with pentostatin. The first 224 patients were treated with cladribine at a dosage of 0.085 mg/kg/d for 7 days by continuous infusion. Subsequent patients received cladribine at a dosage of 0.1 mg/kg/d for 7 days. The overall response rate was 98%, with 91% achieving a complete response. Eight patients did not respond. Fourteen of the 22 partial responders had normalization of their blood counts and spleen size. All of these patients had residual disease in the bone marrow. Seventy-four percent of patients were free of disease progression at 29 months. Four-year overall survival was 96%.

Scripps Clinic investigators have reported on the extended follow-up on 207 patients who were treated with cladribine [26]. All of these patients have been followed for at least 7 years with a median follow-up of 108 months. One hundred and nineteen patients (57%) were untreated previously, 67 patients (32%) had received interferon-α, 45 patients (22%) had undergone splenectomy, and 4 patients had received pentostatin (2%). Overall response rate was 100%; 95% of patients achieved complete remissions and 5% of patients achieved partial remissions. Seventy-six (37%) patients relapsed after their first course of cladribine; the median time to relapse was 42 months. Time to relapse after a partial remission was significantly shorter than after a complete remission (31 months versus 44 months; $P < .0005$). Overall survival of this cohort was 97% at 108 months; however, several patients have required multiple courses of cladribine or other salvage therapies.

The results with cladribine from other institutions are similar to the Scripps Clinic experience. In the Northwestern University series, 52 patients were treated with cladribine at a dosage of 0.1 mg/kg/d by continuous infusion for 7 days. Fifty patients were evaluable for response; 80% of patients achieved a complete response and 18% achieved a partial response with a single course of cladribine. Responses were durable with 72% being free of disease progression at 4 years. Overall survival was 86% at 4 years. This series also had 1 patient who did not respond initially but who later achieved a complete remission at 6 months. Several of the partial responders were treated with second courses of cladribine. Three of these patients achieved a complete remission. Overall complete remission rate at 6 months was 86% [27]. The same investigators recently updated their experience with 86 consecutive patients who had HCL. Overall response rate was 100%; 79% of patients achieved complete remissions, and 21% achieved partial remissions. Overall survival and progression-free survival at 12 years were 87% and 54%, respectively [28].

Hoffman and colleagues [29] from Long Island Jewish Medical Center treated 49 patients who had HCL. Cladribine was the initial therapy for 21 of the patients, whereas the remainder had undergone splenectomy, interferon, or both. Seventy-six percent of the patients achieved a complete remission and 24% achieved a partial remission. Again, responses were durable. Progression-free survival was 80% after a median follow-up of 55 months. Overall survival was 95%. Four of the patients with a CD25-negative phenotype achieved a partial response and subsequently relapsed.

Several centers outside of the United States also have studied cladribine in HCL. Dearden and colleagues [30] from the Royal Marsden Hospital in the United Kingdom treated 45 patients with a continuous 7-day infusion of cladribine at 0.1 mg/kg/d. Twenty-two patients had received pentostatin, 6 had received interferon-α, and 12 were untreated. Overall response rate was 100%. Eighty-four percent of these patients achieved complete responses, whereas the remainder had partial responses. Median time to relapse was 23.5 months. The investigators also reviewed their experience with pentostatin in the same report. Response rates were virtually identical; however, there were three nonresponders in the group that received pentostatin. The groups that received pentostatin and cladribine were compared although this was not a formal randomized trial. Median time to relapse was longer with pentostatin (51.5 months versus 23.5 months); however, time to relapse was the same when patients who had not been treated previously were compared. Patients who achieved a complete response with either therapy had a 97% overall survival at 5 years. A randomized phase III trial has not been conducted to compare cladribine with pentostatin.

Other European centers have reported excellent success with cladribine in HCL. Jehn and colleagues [31] from Germany recently reported on a 12-year follow-up. This study included 44 patients who were treated with continuous infusion cladribine. Eleven patients had undergone splenectomy, interferon, pentostatin, or a combination of these modalities. Overall response rate was 100%; 98% of patients achieved a complete response. Two of the patients' disease was refractory to pentostatin. Seventeen patients relapsed after cladribine. Overall survival at 12 years was 79%.

Italian investigators have studied alternative dosing schedules of cladribine in HCL. Zinzani and colleagues [32] administered cladribine, as a 2-hour infusion at a dosage of 0.14 mg/kg/d for five consecutive days, to 21 patients. A second group of 16 patients was treated with a weekly 2-hour infusion of 0.14 mg/kg for five consecutive weeks. None of these patients had received previous treatment for HCL. Overall response rate was 100%; 81% of patients achieved a complete remission. Response rates were similar in both groups. Eight patients have relapsed. The relapse rate was similar in both groups. Overall survival at 13 years was 96%. The daily administration schedule induced grade 3 or 4 neutropenia in 72% of the patients, whereas the weekly schedule induced grade 3 or 4 neutropenia in 38% of patients. The incidence of severe thrombocytopenia was similar in the two groups. Table 2 summarizes the published clinical data of cladribine in HCL.

PREDICTORS OF RELAPSE FOLLOWING CLADRIBINE THERAPY

Investigators from Scripps Clinic have examined baseline predictors of relapse following cladribine therapy [26]. Five baseline variables (disease duration, baseline white blood cell count, baseline hemoglobin concentration, CD103 staining, and baseline platelet count) were examined with a multivariate proportional hazards regression model. Shorter disease duration, higher baseline white blood cell count, and lower baseline hemoglobin concentration were all significant predictors of relapse at the .05 level in multivariate analysis.

Investigators at Northwestern University in Chicago also examined bone marrow biopsies in morphologic complete responders for evidence of minimal residual disease (MRD) following cladribine therapy [33]. Immunostains for CD20, CD45RO, and DBA.44 were used to examine bone marrow sections for MRD. They stained bone marrow biopsies of 39 patients who were treated

Table 2
Cladribine in hairy cell leukemia

Investigators	N	CR	PR	Minor or none
Zinzani et al [32]	37	30	7	0
Jehn et al [31]	44	43	1	0
Hoffman et al [29]	49	37	12	0
Tallman et al [27]	50	40	9	1
Dearden et al [30]	45	38	7	0
Saven et al [25]	349	319	22	8
TOTAL	574	507 (88%)	58 (10%)	9 (2%)

Abbreviations: CR, complete remission; PR, partial remission.

with cladribine and 27 patients who were treated with pentostatin; 5 and 7 patients had detectable MRD in the bone marrow specimens, respectively. Relapse rate among patients who had MRD was 50%. Only 6% of patients who did not have MRD relapsed. Patients who did not have MRD had a prolonged relapse-free survival compared with patients who had MRD. Four-year relapse-free survival was 55% in patients who had MRD and 88% in patients who did not have MRD ($P = 0.0023$).

RETREATMENT WITH CLADRIBINE UPON RELAPSE
The 7-year follow-up from Scripps Clinic that was reported by Goodman and colleagues [26] included 59 patients who had received a second course of cladribine upon relapse. High response rates were achieved with second infusion of cladribine (Table 3). Seventy-five percent of the patients achieved a complete response and 17% achieved a partial response. There were five (8%) nonresponders. Median response duration was 35 months. Twenty patients suffered a second relapse; 10 of these patients received a third course of cladribine. Once again high response rates were achieved: 60% obtained a complete remission and 20% achieved a partial remission. In this series, 2 patients received a fourth infusion of cladribine; one patient was evaluable and remains in complete remission at 42 months.

In the Northwestern University series, 23 patients who had relapsed HCL were treated with a second infusion of cladribine. The results were similar to those from the Scripps Clinic. The complete response rate to the second cladribine infusion was 52%; with a further 30% achieving a partial remission [28].

TOXICITIES AND COMPLICATIONS OF CLADRIBINE THERAPY
The primary toxicity of cladribine therapy is bone marrow suppression. The initial phase I dose escalation studies were performed in patients who underwent bone marrow transplantation. Severe myelosuppression was seen at a dosage of 0.4 mg/kg/d given by continuous infusion for 10 to 14 days when given in combination with cyclophosphamide and total body irradiation. This dosage also caused severe renal and central nervous system toxicity; several of these patients required hemodialysis. These toxicities were irreversible in several patients. The neurotoxicity was manifested as demyelination. The contribution of cladribine to these toxicities is not clear [6].

Table 3
Selected studies of cladribine retreatment upon relapse

Investigators	Relapse	N	CR (%)	PR (%)	NR/NE (%)	Median response
Goodman et al [26]	#1	59	44 (75)	10 (17)	5 (8)	35 mo
	#2	9	6 (67)	2 (22)	1 (11)	20 mo
	#3	2	1 (50)	0 (0)	1 (50)	42+ mo
Chadha et al [28]	#1	23	12 (52)	7 (30)	4 (18)	Not reported

Abbreviations: CR, complete remission; PR, partial remission.

Dose escalation studies established a maximal tolerated dose (MTD) of 0.1 mg/kg/d by continuous infusion for 7 days. Daily infusion of 0.085 to 0.1 mg/kg/d for 7 days does not cause alopecia, renal toxicity, liver toxicity, nausea, emesis, neurotoxicity, or cardiac problems. Single courses of cladribine caused temporary bone marrow suppression that was manifested by neutropenia and thrombocytopenia. Repeated courses can cause prolonged thrombocytopenia and neutropenia, which often last for longer than 6 months [16].

The principal acute complication of cladribine in HCL is neutropenic fever. Myelosuppression was the major toxicity in the Scripps Clinic series, with 97% of the patients developing grade 3 or 4 neutropenia [25]. The prevalence of temperature greater than 38.5°C was 42%; however, infections were documented in only 13% of these patients. Bacterial infections were most common. Gram-positive infections were more common than were gram-negative infections. Ten patients also had documented viral infections. No fungal infections were reported.

Scripps Clinic investigators also studied the use of filgrastim to decrease the incidence of neutropenia and neutropenic fever in patients who had HCL and were treated with cladribine and compared the results to historic controls treated with cladribine alone [34]. Thirty-five patients received filgrastim at 5 µg/kg/d subcutaneously on days −1, −2, and −3 before receiving the standard infusion of cladribine. Filgrastim was administered again after the infusion was completed, and continued until the ANC was greater than 2×10^9/L on two consecutive days. Filgrastim increased the nadir ANC from 0.22×10^9/L to 0.53×10^9/L ($P = .04$). It also decreased the time to achievement of an ANC of greater than 1.0×10^9/L from 22 days to 9 days. The percentage of febrile patients, number of febrile days, and frequency of admissions for antibiotics was not different between the two groups. Therefore, the routine adjunctive use of filgrastim in cladribine treatment of HCL is not recommended.

Cladribine causes prolonged lymphocytopenia. The $CD4^+$ T-cell subset is decreased for the longest duration [35]; however, cladribine affects B and T lymphocytes [6,36]. Cladribine also inhibits B- and T-cell activation in vitro [15,37]. Lymphocytopenia may contribute to the increased risk for delayed opportunistic infections. In the Scripps Clinic series, five patients developed herpes zoster, which was the most common delayed infection. Two patients had positive hepatitis C serology, but both patients had received blood transfusions previously. Two patients were diagnosed with mycobacterial infections, one each with *Mycobacterium tuberculosis* and *M chelonei* [25].

The Scripps Clinic investigators also reported a 20% prevalence of grade 3 and 4 thrombocytopenia. There was a 22% prevalence of grade 3 and 4 anemia [25]. Cheson and colleagues [38] reported the rare complication of hemolysis in cladribine treatment of HCL. Two of 895 patients developed hemolytic anemia; both cases resolved and were not considered to be life threatening.

In the extended follow-up of the Scripps Clinics' patients who had HCL that was reported by Goodman and colleagues [26], 47 of the 208 evaluable patients developed 58 second malignancies (Table 4). This represented a twofold increase over the National Cancer Institute Surveillance Epidemiology and

Table 4
Second malignancies in hairy cell leukemia

Investigators	N	Previous treatment	Observed expected ratio	No. of second malignancies (%)	Comments
Au et al [39]	117	All	2.60	36 (31%)	Increased risk, not therapy related
Kurzrock et al [40]	350	All	1.34	26 (7%)	Increased myeloma/ lymphoma risk, not therapy related
Goodman et al [26]	379	Cladribine	2.03	47 (12%)	Slight increased risk
Chadha et al [28]	86	Cladribine	Not reported	15 (17%)	

End Result database. Most patients had a previous diagnosis of a second malignancy. Statistical analysis identified advanced age as a risk factor for a second malignancy. Patients with a history of second malignancy had a hazard ratio of 3.70, whereas elderly patients had a hazard ratio of 2.03. The most common second malignancy was nonmelanoma skin cancer. Seventeen patients developed 20 nonmelanoma skin cancers. Fourteen patients developed adenocarcinoma of the prostate. Three patients developed secondary non-Hodgkin's lymphoma. Colon, breast, renal cell, gastric, and hepatocellular carcinomas also were recorded.

Au and colleagues [39] reported on the incidence of second malignancies in patients who had HCL from British Columbia, Canada. There was an increased incidence of second malignancies when compared with normal, age-matched controls. Patients who were treated with a combination of interferon and purine analogs had a more than twofold increase in second malignancies. There were 19 second malignancies in the 67 patients in this series who received cladribine.

Investigators at MD Anderson Cancer Center reported on 350 patients who had HCL and described the incidence of second malignancies [40]. Twenty-six patients developed second malignancies. Although there was an increased incidence of second malignancies, it did not reach statistical significance when compared with standardized incidence ratios from the Connecticut Tumor Registry. These patients had been treated with cladribine, pentostatin, or interferon-α. There was no increase in solid tumors with any of the three agents; however, there was an 8.7-fold increase in lymphoid neoplasms ($P = .03$) and a 13.04-fold increase in myeloma-related neoplasms ($P < .001$).

SALVAGE TREATMENTS FOLLOWING CLADRIBINE
Rituximab
Rituximab is a monoclonal antibody that is directed against the B-cell antigen CD20. Hagberg [41] first published a case report in 1999 of a patient who had HCL and achieved a complete response following rituximab. Previously, this patient had obtained a partial response and subsequently relapsed following

cladribine therapy. Italian investigators then published their experience with 10 patients who had relapsed HCL who received rituximab, 375 mg/m^2/wk for 4 weeks. Overall response rate was 50%; 40% of patients achieved a partial remission and 10% achieved a complete remission [42]. Nieva and colleagues [43] at Scripps Clinic also conducted a phase II study of rituximab in the salvage setting following a cladribine relapse. Twenty-four patients who had relapsed HCL were treated with four weekly dosages of rituximab, 375 mg/m^2/wk. Overall response rate was 25%. Three patients achieved a partial remission and 3 others patients achieved a complete remission. Rituximab was tolerated well in all of the studies.

Interferon-α

Interferon-α has in vitro activity against hairy cells. It induces apoptosis of non-adherent hairy cells in culture by increasing tumor necrosis factor-α production and increasing hairy cell sensitivity to tumor necrosis factor-α [44]. It represents a modestly effective salvage therapy for some patients who relapsed after treatment with cladribine, although it only has been evaluated in small numbers of patients. Scripps Clinic investigators treated nine patients who had HCL with interferon-α after they relapsed following treatment with cladribine. One patient achieved a complete response, 2 patients achieved a partial response, and 6 patients did not respond [25].

Seymour and colleagues [45] treated three patients who had HCL with interferon-α after they relapsed following treatment with cladribine. All three achieved a response, which was maintained while on therapy. Two of the three patients relapsed when the interferon-α was discontinued.

BL-22 Immunotoxin

Classic and variant HCL commonly express CD22 on their cell surface. BL22 is an immunotoxin that binds to CD22 and is conjugated to a pseudomonas exotoxin. Kreitman and colleagues [46] conducted a dose escalation trial of BL22 in patients who had B-cell malignancies. Sixteen of the 31 patients enrolled had HCL. All 16 had failed cladribine, and the median number of treatments was three. Eleven of the 16 patients achieved a complete response, and 2 patients achieved a partial response. Three of the 11 patients who achieved complete remission relapsed, but achieved a second complete remission upon retreatment. The hemolytic uremic syndrome is an unusual and potentially life-threatening complication of BL-22 immunotoxin, and was documented in two patients at the National Institutes of Health. They were treated with plasmapheresis, did not require dialysis, and the syndrome resolved completely in both patients who achieved a complete response.

Pentostatin

Pentostatin is a purine nucleoside analog that acts as a direct and irreversible inhibitor of ADA. Treatment with pentostatin results in the intracellular accumulation of deoxyadenosine triphosphate, which causes apoptosis.

Pentostatin is administered at 4 mg/m^2 every other week for 3 to 6 months. It is potently immunosuppressive, especially in patients with diminished renal function, the elderly, and those with poor bone marrow reserve [47,48]. Patients who have disease that is refractory to cladribine or who relapsed after treatment with cladribine may respond to pentostatin, and vice versa [25,49]. This is despite mechanistic similarities between the two drugs. Scripps Clinic investigators treated seven patients who had failed cladribine therapy with pentostatin. Three patients achieved complete responses, three had partial responses, and one failed to respond. Pentostatin likely represents a rational treatment after cladribine in relapsed or resistant patients; however, there are no large controlled studies to address this subgroup of patients that has relapsed HCL.

Splenectomy

Current indications for splenectomy include chemotherapy failure, active or uncontrolled infections, symptomatic or ruptured splenomegaly, or bleeding that is associated with severe thrombocytopenia. In the Scripps Clinic series, one patient who was resistant to cladribine was treated with splenectomy with improvement in his cytopenias. Two other patients, who relapsed after an initial response, were treated with splenectomy; neither patient derived benefit from this surgical procedure [25].

Stem Cell Transplantation

Few patients who have HCL have undergone high-dose chemotherapy with stem cell rescue. Cheever and colleagues [50] reported the treatment of a patient who had HCL with high-dose chemoradiotherapy followed by a syngeneic bone marrow transplant. This patient experienced a prolonged complete response.

One patient, who had failed multiple treatments, including cladribine, underwent a nonmyeloablative allogeneic stem cell transplant at Scripps Clinic (unpublished data). He has experienced a prolonged disease-free survival.

Alemtuzumab

Hairy cells strongly express CD52. Alemtuzumab is a monoclonal anti-CD52 antibody that has activity in chronic lymphocytic leukemia [51]. Because hairy cells express CD52, this represents a rational therapeutic approach.

SUMMARY

Cladribine results in prolonged complete remissions in most patients who have HCL. Several studies have indicated that patients who are in complete remission have survivals that are comparable to those of normal age-matched controls. HCL-related mortality is distinctly uncommon. Nevertheless, it is unlikely that cladribine treatment of HCL is curative because MRD is common in the bone marrows of complete responders. Response criteria for HCL include clinical, hematologic, and morphologic criteria, but do not include flow cytometry, immunohistochemical analysis, or molecular studies. More sensitive techniques have been used by Filleul and colleagues [52] to detect MRD. They used clonogenic probes from the hypervariable regions of the immunoglobulin heavy-chain gene and performed polymerase chain reactions (PCRs) on bone marrow biopsy specimens. All seven patients who were in morphologic complete remission after a single cladribine infusion were PCR positive.

These data indicate that cladribine induces protracted remissions but is not necessarily curative. MRD can be detected in most patients when sensitive techniques are used. Persistence of immunohistochemical MRD may predict a higher likelihood for clinical relapse. The clinical significance of PCR-detected MRD remains to be studied in a large number of patients.

Investigators from the University of Pisa in Italy have used a combination of cladribine and rituximab to eradicate MRD in patients who have HCL. Ten patients received treatment with a standard infusion of cladribine. Two patients achieved a complete remission, 6 patients achieved a partial remission, and 2 patients failed to respond. All were PCR positive for the immunoglobulin heavy-chain (IgH) gene product at the completion of cladribine treatment. All 10 patients received four weekly treatments of rituximab, 375 mg/m²/wk. Eight patients who were evaluable for molecular response became IgH PCR negative 12 months after the completion of rituximab therapy. All 10 patients had achieved a complete hematologic response 2 months after the completion of rituximab therapy [53]. The curative nature of this treatment will require long-term follow-up.

Cladribine represents a major therapeutic advance in the treatment of HCL. The prognosis of patients who have HCL has been improved greatly with cladribine therapy. Future strategies should address combination therapy with purine analogs and monoclonal antibodies. These strategies should address eradication of MRD in an attempt to develop a potentially curative combination treatment program.

References

[1] Jansen J, Hermans J. Splenectomy in hairy cell leukemia: a retrospective multicenter analysis. Cancer 1981;47(8):2066–76.

[2] Mintz U, Golomb HM. Splenectomy as initial therapy in twenty-six patients with leukemic reticuloendotheliosis (hairy cell leukemia). Cancer Res 1979;39(7 Pt 1):2366–70.

[3] Giblett ER, Anderson JE, Cohen F, et al. Adenosine-deaminase deficiency in two patients with severely impaired cellular immunity. Lancet 1972;2(7786):1067–9.

[4] Cohen A, Hirschhorn R, Horowitz SD, et al. Deoxyadenosine triphosphate as a potentially toxic metabolite in adenosine deaminase deficiency. Proc Natl Acad Sci U S A 1978;75(1): 472–6.

[5] Carson DA, Kaye J, Seegmiller JE. Lymphospecific toxicity in adenosine deaminase deficiency and purine nucleoside phosphorylase deficiency: possible role of nucleoside kinase(s). Proc Natl Acad Sci U S A 1977;74(12):5677–81.

[6] Beutler E. Cladribine (2-chlorodeoxyadenosine). Lancet 1992;340(8825):952–6.

[7] Carson DA, Wasson DB, Kaye J, et al. Deoxycytidine kinase-mediated toxicity of deoxyadenosine analogs toward malignant human lymphoblasts in vitro and toward murine L1210 leukemia in vivo. Proc Natl Acad Sci U S A 1980;77(11):6865–9.

[8] Carson DA, Kaye J, Seegmiller JE. Differential sensitivity of human leukemic T cell lines and B cell lines to growth inhibition by deoxyadenosine. J Immunol 1978;121(5):1726–31.

[9] Leoni LM, Chao Q, Cottam HB, et al. Induction of an apoptotic program in cell-free extracts by 2-chloro-2′-deoxyadenosine 5′-triphosphate and cytochrome c. Proc Natl Acad Sci U S A 1998;95(16):9567–71.

[10] Genini D, Budihardjo I, Plunkett W, et al. Nucleotide requirements for the in vitro activation of the apoptosis protein-activating factor-1-mediated caspase pathway. J Biol Chem 2000;275(1):29–34.

[11] Carson DA, Seto S, Wasson DB, et al. DNA strand breaks, NAD metabolism, and programmed cell death. Exp Cell Res 1986;164(2):273–81.

[12] Robertson LE, Chubb S, Meyn RE, et al. Induction of apoptotic cell death in chronic lymphocytic leukemia by 2-chloro-2′-deoxyadenosine and 9-beta-D-arabinosyl-2-fluoroadenine. Blood 1993;81(1):143–50.

[13] Carrera CJ, Terai C, Lotz M, et al. Potent toxicity of 2-chlorodeoxyadenosine toward human monocytes in vitro and in vivo. A novel approach to immunosuppressive therapy. J Clin Invest 1990;86(5):1480–8.

[14] Christensen LF, Brown AD, Robins MJ, et al. Synthesis and biological activity of selected 2, 6 di-substituted (2-deoxy-α and β-D-erythro-pentofuranosyl) purines. J Med Chem 1975;15:735–9.

[15] Liliemark J, Juliusson G. On the pharmacokinetics of 2-chloro-2′-deoxyadenosine in humans. Cancer Res 1991;51(20):5570–2.

[16] Carson DA, Wasson DB, Beutler E. Antileukemic and immunosuppressive activity of 2-chloro-2′-deoxyadenosine. Proc Natl Acad Sci U S A 1984;81(7):2232–6.

[17] Carson DA, Wasson DB, Esparza LM, et al. Oral antilymphocyte activity and induction of apoptosis by 2-chloro-2′-arabino-fluoro-2′-deoxyadenosine. Proc Natl Acad Sci U S A 1992;89(7):2970–4.

[18] Saven A, Carrera CJ, Carson DA, et al. 2-Chlorodeoxyadenosine treatment of refractory chronic lymphocytic leukemia. Leuk Lymphoma 1991;5(Suppl):133–8.

[19] Juliusson G, Heldal D, Hippe E, et al. Subcutaneous injections of 2-chlorodeoxyadenosine for symptomatic hairy cell leukemia. J Clin Oncol 1995;13(4):989–95.

[20] Lauria F, Bocchia M, Marotta G, et al. Weekly administration of 2-chlorodeoxyadenosine in patients with hairy cell leukemia: A new treatment schedule effective and safer in preventing infectious complications [letter]. Blood 1998;89:1838–9.

[21] Saven A, Cheung WK, Smith I, et al. Pharmacokinetic study of oral and bolus intravenous 2-chlorodeoxyadenosine in patients with malignancy. J Clin Oncol 1996;14(3):978–83.

[22] Parsons PG, Bowman EPW, Blakley RC. Selective toxicity of deoxyadenosine analogues in human melanoma cell lines. Biochem Pharmacol 1986;65:4025–9.

[23] Carrera CJ, Piro LD, Miller WE, et al. Remission induction in hairy cell leukemia by treatment with 2-chlorodeoxyadenosine: Role of DNA strand breaks and NAD depletion [abstract]. Clin Res 1987;35:597A.

[24] Piro LD, Carrera CJ, Carson DA, et al. Lasting remissions in hairy-cell leukemia induced by a single infusion of 2-chlorodeoxyadenosine. N Engl J Med 1990;322(16):1117–21.

[25] Saven A, Burian C, Koziol JA, et al. Long-term follow-up of patients with hairy cell leukemia after cladribine treatment. Blood 1998;92(6):1918–26.

[26] Goodman GR, Burian C, Koziol JA, et al. Extended follow-up of patients with hairy cell leukemia after treatment with cladribine. J Clin Oncol 2003;21:891–6.

[27] Tallman MS, Hakimian D, Rademaker AW, et al. Relapse of hairy cell leukemia after 2-chlorodeoxyadenosine: long-term follow-up of the Northwestern University experience. Blood 1996;88(6):1954–9.

[28] Chadha P, Rademaker AW, Mendiratta P, et al. Treatment of hairy cell leukemia with 2-chlorodeoxyadenosine (2-CdA): long-term follow-up of the Northwestern University experience. Blood 2005;106(1):241–6.

[29] Hoffman MA, Janson D, Rose E, et al. Treatment of hairy-cell leukemia with cladribine: response, toxicity, and long-term follow-up. J Clin Oncol 1997;15(3):1138–42.

[30] Dearden CE, Matutes E, Hilditch BL, et al. Long-term follow-up of patients with hairy cell leukemia after treatment with pentostatin or cladribine. Br J Haematol 1999;106(2):515–9.

[31] Jehn U, Bartl R, Dietzfelbinger H, et al. An update: 12-year follow-up of patients with hairy cell leukemia following treatment with 2-chlorodeoxyadenosine. Leukemia 2004;18(9):1476–81.

[32] Zinzani PL, Tani M, Marchi E, et al. Long-term follow-up of front-line treatment of hairy cell leukemia with 2-chlorodeoxyadenosine. Haematologica 2004;89(3):309–13.

[33] Tallman MS, Hakimian D, Kopecky KJ, et al. Minimal residual disease in patients with hairy cell leukemia in complete remission treated with 2-chlorodeoxyadenosine or 2-deoxycoformycin and prediction of early relapse. Clin Cancer Res 1999;5(7):1665–70.

[34] Saven A, Burian C, Adusumalli J, et al. Filgrastim for cladribine-induced neutropenic fever in patients with hairy cell leukemia. Blood 1999;93(8):2471–7.

[35] Seymour JF, Kurzrock R, Freireich EJ, et al. 2-chlorodeoxyadenosine induces durable remissions and prolonged suppression of CD4$^+$ lymphocyte counts in patients with hairy cell leukemia. Blood 1994;83(10):2906–11.

[36] Saven A, Piro LD. 2-Chlorodeoxyadenosine: a newer purine analog active in the treatment of indolent lymphoid malignancies. Ann Intern Med 1994;120(9):784–91.

[37] Gorski A, Grieb P, Korczak-Kowalska G, et al. Cladribine (2-chloro-deoxyadenosine, CDA): an inhibitor of human B and T cell activation in vitro. Immunopharmacology 1993;26(3):197–202.

[38] Cheson BD, Sorensen JM, Vena DA, et al. Treatment of hairy cell leukemia with 2-chlorodeoxyadenosine via the Group C protocol mechanism of the National Cancer Institute: a report of 979 patients. J Clin Oncol 1998;16(9):3007–15.

[39] Au WY, Klasa RJ, Gallagher R, et al. Second malignancies in patients with hairy cell leukemia in British Columbia: a 20-year experience. Blood 1998;92:1160–4.

[40] Kurzrock R, Strom SS, Estey E, et al. Second cancer risk in hairy cell leukemia: analysis of 350 patients. J Clin Oncol 1997;15(5):1803–10.

[41] Hagberg H. Chimeric monoclonal anti-CD20 antibody (rituximab)—an effective treatment for a patient with relapsing hairy cell leukaemia. Med Oncol 1999;16(3):221–2.

[42] Lauria F, Lenoci M, Annino L, et al. Efficacy of anti-CD20 monoclonal antibodies (Mabthera) in patients with progressed hairy cell leukemia. Haematologica 2001;86(10):1046–50.

[43] Nieva J, Bethel K, Saven A. Phase 2 study of rituximab in the treatment of cladribine-failed patients with hairy cell leukemia. Blood 2003;102(3):810–3.

[44] Baker PK, Pettitt AR, Slupsky JR, et al. Response of hairy cells to IFN-alpha involves induction of apoptosis through autocrine TNF-alpha and protection by adhesion. Blood 2002;100(2):647–53.

[45] Seymour JF, Estey EH, Keating MJ, et al. Response to interferon-α in patients with hairy cell leukemia relapsing after treatment with 2-chlorodeoxyadenosine. Leukemia 1995;9:929–32.

[46] Kreitman RJ, Wilson WH, Bergeron K, et al. Efficacy of the anti-CD22 recombinant immunotoxin BL22 in chemotherapy-resistant hairy-cell leukemia. N Engl J Med 2001;345(4):241–7.

[47] Cassileth PA, Cheuvart B, Spiers AS, et al. Pentostatin induces durable remissions in hairy cell leukemia. J Clin Oncol 1991;9(2):243–6.

[48] Ho AD, Thaler J, Stryckmans P, et al. Pentostatin in refractory chronic lymphocytic leukemia: a phase II trial of the European Organization for Research and Treatment of Cancer. J Natl Cancer Inst 1990;82(17):1416–20.

[49] Saven A, Piro LD. Complete remissions in hairy cell leukemia with 2-chlorodeoxyadenosine after failure with 2'-deoxycoformycin. Ann Intern Med 1993;119(4):278–83.

[50] Cheever MA, Fefer A, Greenberg PD, et al. Treatment of hairy-cell leukemia with chemoradiotherapy and identical twin bone-marrow transplantation. N Engl J Med 1982;307(8):479–81.

[51] Moreton P, Kennedy B, Lucas G, et al. Eradication of minimal residual disease in B-cell chronic lymphocytic leukemia after alemtuzumab therapy is associated with prolonged survival. J Clin Oncol 2005;23(13):2971–9.

[52] Filleul B, Delannoy A, Ferrant A, et al. A single course of 2-chloro-deoxyadenosine does not eradicate leukemic cells in hairy cell leukemia patients in complete remission. Leukemia 1994;8(7):1153–6.

[53] Cervetti G, Galimberti S, Andreazzoli F, et al. Rituximab as treatment for minimal residual disease in hairy cell leukaemia. Eur J Haematol 2004;73(6):412–7.

HEMATOLOGY/ONCOLOGY CLINICS
OF NORTH AMERICA

.SEVIER
∧UNDERS

Monoclonal Antibody Therapy for Hairy Cell Leukemia

Deborah A. Thomas, MD*, Farhad Ravandi, MD,
Hagop Kantarjian, MD

Department of Leukemia, University of Texas M.D. Anderson Cancer Center, 1515 Holcombe
Boulevard, Unit 428, Houston, TX 77030, USA

Hairy cell leukemia (HCL) is an uncommon indolent B-lineage lymphoid neoplasm that is characterized by infiltration of the bone marrow, liver, spleen, and occasionally lymph nodes, which results in a typical presentation of pancytopenia and splenomegaly [1]. The cell of origin of HCL remains to be elucidated. Initially, it was surmised that HCL results from clonal expansion of mature B cells with light-chain–restricted surface immunoglobulin (Ig) expression [2]. The unusual expression of multiple Ig heavy-chain isotypes with a predominance of IgG3 was noted [3]. Investigators also demonstrated that multiple clonally related isotypes could be observed within individual hairy cells, which suggested generation of these isotypes by way of RNA splicing [4]. Thus, it was postulated that hairy cells are arrested at a stage of isotype switching with RNA processing that precedes deletional recombinations [5]. Mutated Ig heavy-chain variable gene (IgHv) also is expressed in most cases of HCL, which suggests an origin from a postgerminal center antigen-exposed memory B cell [5,6]. Gene expression profiling has failed to differentiate subsets of HCL, and profiles most often resemble those of memory B cells [7].

Immunophenotypic expression of the B-cell associated antigens CD19, CD20, CD22, FMC-7, and CD79a, as well as the antigens CD11c, CD103, and CD25 are characteristic of HCL [8,9]. CD52 expression also has been reported in most cases studied [10]. Such characteristic immunophenotypic expression profiles aid in the detection of minimal residual disease (MRD) in HCL by the use of multi-parameter flow cytometry techniques. Flow cytometry seems more sensitive and specific than polymerase chain reaction (PCR) assays for IgH for the detection of MRD after therapy [11].

The efficacy of frontline treatment with single-agent nucleoside analog therapy (eg, 2-chlorodeoxyadenosine [2-CdA] or deoxycoformycin) has been confirmed by several investigators, with complete remission (CR) rates of 80% to 90% [12–17]. Four- to 5-year progression-free survival rates range from 70% to 85% after one or two courses of 2-CdA; with extended follow-up, these rates

*Corresponding author. E-mail address: debthomas@mdanderson.org (D.A. Thomas).

0889-8588/06/$ – see front matter
doi:10.1016/j.hoc.2006.06.011

decrease to 50% to 60% without a plateau in the curve [18–20]. Although the overall survival rates of 85% to 90% after nucleoside analog therapy are favorable, the increasing proportion of recurrences observed with longer follow-up suggests that such therapy may not be sufficient to eradicate HCL. Predictors of treatment failure include baseline features such as lower hemoglobin level, higher leukocyte count, and shorter disease duration prior to initiation of therapy. Achievement of partial response (PR) compared with CR after nucleoside analog therapy also portends a higher likelihood of disease recurrence [18,21].

RELAPSED OR REFRACTORY HAIRY CELL LEUKEMIA

Approximately 25% to 40% of patients who have HCL relapse within 3 to 5 years after undergoing nucleoside analog therapy [18–20]. Treatment of relapsed or refractory HCL is not standardized. Therapy options include splenectomy [22], interferon-α [23–25], retreatment with nucleoside analogs [18,26], immunotoxin therapy (eg, anti-CD22 conjugated to the *Pseudomonas* exotoxin or BL-22 [27,28]), tumor necrosis factor-α inhibitors, angiogenesis inhibitors, and monoclonal antibody (MoAb) therapy. Remission rates after retreatment with the nucleoside analogs range from 70% to 90%, but responses often are not durable [15,18,26,29]. In addition, the repetitive administration of nucleoside analog therapy can be associated with prolonged CD4 lymphopenia, bone marrow aplasia with cytopenias that require transfusion support, and potentially serious opportunistic infections related to the prolonged immunosuppression or myelosuppression [30–34].

PRINCIPLES OF MONOCLONAL ANTIBODY THERAPY

Ideally, the target antigen should be expressed on nearly all of the malignant cells with minimal or no expression on normal cells. Alternatively, if normal cells express the antigen, antibody-mediated elimination of these cells should not have significant clinical consequences. The aim of the antibody should be to induce cell death by (1) neutralizing the effect of a growth factor, which induces apoptosis, (2) activation of effector mechanisms of the host (such as complement activation), or (3) cytotoxicity that is directed against effector cells, such as macrophages or natural killer cells by way of interaction with cellular receptors for IgG (Fcγ receptors; FcγRs). The Fc portions of the MoAb's seem to be a major component of the therapeutic activity. Polymorphisms of FcγRIIIb (Val/Phe^{158}) and FcγRIIa (His/Arg^{131}) affect binding of the IgG–immune complexes, and, thus, affect efficacy. Modulation of the antigen and potential shedding into plasma may decrease efficacy if associated with decreased surface expression and neutralization of the MoAb by complexing with soluble forms [35].

The MoAb should be accessible to the sites of disease activity. For example, the anti-CD52 MoAb alemtuzumab has superior efficacy in eradicating disease in the peripheral blood, spleen, and bone marrow compartments compared with lymph nodes (reduced efficacy for bulky lymphadenopathy). This makes it an attractive agent to study systematically in HCL, because lymphadenopathy rarely is a manifestation of the disease [36,37]. Other target antigens include CD20, CD22, and CD25; all are expressed highly in HCL [38]. Several MoAb's that target these antigens are of interest for the treatment of HCL.

RITUXIMAB IN PREVIOUSLY TREATED HAIRY CELL LEUKEMIA

Rituximab is a high-affinity chimeric MoAb that is directed against CD20, a pan–B-cell antigen that is expressed highly on the surface of hairy cells (eg, 312 ± 10^9/L CD20 molecules per HCL cell compared with 65 ± 10^9/L per cell for chronic lymphocytic leukemia [CLL]) [9]. The CD20 antigen is a human B lymphocyte–restricted differentiation phosphoprotein that is located on pre-B and mature B lymphocytes and indolent non-Hodgkin's lymphomas (NHLs) [39–41]. The antibody is an IgG1 κ immunoglobulin that contains murine light- and heavy-chain variable region sequences and human constant region sequences. Rituximab directly induces apoptosis in addition to complement- and antibody-mediated cellular cytotoxicity (ADCC) [40,42,43]. It demonstrated significant activity as a single agent in previously treated low-grade NHL with standard dosing of 375 mg/m^2 for four weekly doses [44,45]. An improvement in the response rate was observed with extended dosing (8 weeks) in previously treated low-grade NHL [46].

Initial trials of rituximab in CLL were disappointing; low response rates were attributed to the decreased expression of CD20 compared with low-grade NHL. Clinical trials of dose-escalated or dose-intensive rituximab in relapsed or refractory CLL showed an improvement in the response rates; however, most were PRs [47,48]. Soluble CD20 later was shown to be detectable in the plasma of patients who had CLL, and higher levels seemed to correlate with worse outcome [49]. This suggested that pharmacologic monitoring of rituximab levels and soluble CD20 levels might be needed to direct single-agent therapy.

Several clinical trials of single-agent rituximab therapy have been conducted in previously treated HCL (Table 1) [50–53]. Clinical activity also was reported in limited case report series [54–56]. Hagberg and Lundholm [50] reported a response rate of 75% (CR rate of 62%) in eight patients who had previously treated HCL after four standard weekly doses. Lauria and colleagues [51] reported a response rate of 50% (CR rate of 10%) with a similar regimen; however, remission criteria were strict and required negative immunostaining. Nieva and colleagues [52] reported an overall response rate of only 26% (CR rate of 13%) with rituximab. Extended dosing of rituximab for an 8-week course was studied in 15 patients who had previously treated HCL; overall response rate was 80% [53]. Treatment with rituximab generally was tolerated well without undue toxicity in any of these reports. Responses seemed to be durable in most patients who achieved CR, although follow-up in these series was relatively short.

Reasons for the differential activity of rituximab among these clinical trials could include, among other factors (eg, advanced disease status), the dosing schema used (eg, 4 versus 8 weeks of therapy), soluble CD20 expression that resulted in antibody neutralization, or IgG FCγ receptor polymorphisms.

Table 1
Single-agent rituximab therapy in hairy cell leukemia

Study	N	Dosing (mg/m^2)	CR (%)	PR (%)	OR (%)
Lauria et al [51]	10	375 × 4 weeks	10	40	50
Hagberg and Lundholm [50]	11	375 × 4 weeks	55[a]	10	64
Thomas et al [53]	15	375 × 8 weeks	66	13	80
Nieva et al [52]	24	375 × 4 weeks	13	13	26

Abbreviation: OR, overall response.
[a] CR rate was 33% for three untreated patients.

The susceptibility of the hairy cells after exposure to monoclonal antibodies depends on the activation of effector cells by way of their IgG FcγRs. Several FcγR polymorphisms have been identified that may affect the killing function of natural killer cells and macrophages. In a clinical trial of rituximab therapy for indolent NHL, Weng and Levy [57] determined that FcγRIIIa 158 valine/valine and the FcγRIIa 131 histidine/histidine genotypes were associated independently with response rate and freedom from progression. However, in a clinical trial of dose-intensive rituximab in previously treated CLL, FcγRIIIa polymorphisms were not predictive of response, which suggested that, unlike indolent NHL, mechanisms of tumor clearance other than antibody-dependent cellular cytotoxicity may be more important [58]. These polymorphisms have not been studied systematically in HCL. Second-generation anti-CD20 MoAb's (Hu-Max-CD20, GenMab, Inc., Princeton, New Jersey) have been developed, and clinical trials in several lymphoid malignancies are underway [59–61].

RITUXIMAB IN FRONTLINE THERAPY OF HAIRY CELL LEUKEMIA

Detection of MRD by multi-parameter flow cytometry or by PCR for IgH gene rearrangements, was shown by some investigators to be predictive of disease recurrence after nucleoside analog therapy [62–64]. Recent therapeutic approaches that are designed to improve relapse-free survival in HCL have been directed at the eradication of MRD. Several studies have shown synergy between rituximab and several chemotherapeutic agents, including nucleoside analogs [65].

Cervetti and colleagues [66] treated 10 patients with standard-dose rituximab for 4 weeks after demonstrating persistent MRD by PCR for IgH subsequent to one course of 2-CdA therapy. Two patients were in CR, 6 patients had achieved PR, and 2 patients had failed to respond to 2-CdA. All 8 patients achieved CR after treatment with rituximab, as assessed within 2 months after therapy. Sequential assessments of PCR for IgH after rituximab therapy showed reduction in quantitative PCR levels or molecular negativity in several patients; in some cases the latter response was not observed until 12 months after completion of rituximab. Ravandi and colleagues [67] recently reported efficacy of the combination of 2-CdA, 5.6 mg/m^2 intravenously daily by bolus for 5 days, followed by 8 weekly treatments with standard-dose rituximab initiated on day 28 of 2-CdA therapy, in 13 patients who had previously untreated HCL. The CR rate was 100% with eradication of MRD (assessed by multi-parameter flow cytometry and PCR for IgH) in all but 2 patients after completion of the sequential therapy. No additional toxicity was observed with the combination compared with historical experience with 2-CdA alone. Additional follow-up is required to determine the impact of the sequential addition of MoAb to standard nucleoside analog therapy on progression-free survival. Clinical trials that combine nucleoside analogs with rituximab should be considered given the favorable outcomes observed with such combinations for the frontline treatment of CLL [68,69].

ALEMTUZUMAB
Alemtuzumab is a humanized rat IgG1 MoAb that is directed against the CD52 antigen. CD52 expression has been reported in normal cells and several other chronic lymphoid leukemias, including CLL and T-cell prolymphocytic leukemia [70]. Alemtuzumab has been studied extensively in these diseases, and was approved by the US Food and Drug Administration for the treatment of refractory or relapsed CLL [37,71]. The mechanisms of action include cytolysis via complement fixation and ADCC. Alemtuzumab had superior efficacy in eradicating disease in the peripheral blood, spleen, and bone marrow compartments compared with lymph nodes. A soluble form of CD52 has been detected in the plasma of patients who have CLL. This complexes with alemtuzumab, and may reduce its efficacy [35].

CD52 expression recently was reported in HCL (Table 2) [10,72–75]. In the largest series using systematic application of multi-parameter flow cytometry, the CD52 antigen was detected in 92% to 100% of the hairy cells [10]. CD52 staining on hairy cells appeared approximately equal in intensity to normal T lymphocytes. The activity of alemtuzumab in HCL has not been studied systematically. A report of alemtuzumab used for treatment of a patient who had HCL that was refractory to 2-CdA after rituximab therapy (hematologic improvement but intolerant to therapy with subsequent progression of disease) indicated activity [76]. An improvement in transfusion-dependent thrombocytopenia was observed after alemtuzumab, despite persistence of the marrow disease. The activity of alemtuzumab in similar chronic lymphoid diseases indicates that systematic study of this agent as a therapeutic intervention for HCL is warranted.

EPRATUZUMAB
Classic or variant HCL is usually strongly positive for CD22, a 135-kd transmembrane glycoprotein that is a B-lymphocyte–restricted member of the Ig superfamily [8,77]. It is a member of the sialoglycoprotein family of adhesion molecules that regulates B-cell activation and the interaction of B cells with T cells and antigen-presenting cells [78,79]. This antigen is not expressed on

Table 2
CD52 expression in hairy cell leukemia

Study	No. cases	Methodology	Results
Hale et al [72]	1	Flow cytometry	57% expression
Hale et al [73]	10	Immunofluorescence, complement-mediated cell lysis, flow cytometry	70% cases positive
Dyer [74]	5	Flow cytometry	All cases positive
Belov et al [75]	1	Microarray	All cases positive
Quigley et al [10]	10	Flow cytometry	All cases positive

stem cells and is absent in the early stages of B-cell development. Epratuzumab is a complementarity-determining region-grafted, humanized, IgG1 κ version of the murine MoAb [38,80,81]. Unlike rituximab, epratuzumab has not been shown to induce apoptosis or complement-mediated cytotoxicity, but it does have modest ADCC in vitro. The antibody is internalized rapidly after binding to CD22-expressing lymphoma cells [82]. Efficacy was demonstrated in single-agent phase I and II clinical trials in indolent [83] and aggressive [84] NHL. The toxicity profile is similar to rituximab, with predominantly infusional-related side effects. Clinical activity of epratuzumab has not been determined in HCL.

COMBINATION MONOCLONAL ANTIBODY THERAPY

Activity of combination monoclonal therapy regimens has been reported in relapsed or refractory chronic lymphoid leukemias and lymphomas. Most have increased efficacy compared with single agent therapy. Faderl and colleagues [85] reported an overall response rate of 52% after treatment with a combination of rituximab and alemtuzumab in patients who had previously treated CLL (n = 32), prolymphocytic leukemia, or other hematologic malignancies. Leonard and colleagues [86] treated patients who had previously treated indolent and aggressive NHL with concurrent epratuzumab and rituximab. Overall response rates were in excess of 60% in each histologic subtype. Acceptable toxicity profiles were observed with these regimens, indicating that these therapeutic approaches may warrant further study in HCL.

CYTOKINE MODULATION

Several cytokines have been reported to up regulate the expression of CD20 in CLL [87]. Although there is a high overall expression of CD20 in HCL, there may be marked heterogeneity in the intensity of expression among the individual hairy cells. Thus, augmentation of this target antigen may increase the efficacy of MoAb therapy. Venugopal and colleagues [87] showed an increase in CD20 expression on the surface of CLL cells after exposure to IL-4, granulocyte-macrophage colony-stimulating factor (GM-CSF), and tumor necrosis factor-α. Preclinical in vivo animal studies demonstrated the increased efficacy of rituximab when given in combination with granulocyte colony-stimulating factor or with GM-CSF [88,89]. Ongoing clinical trials of rituximab in combination with GM-CSF in previously treated CLL or indolent NHL demonstrated increased response rates compared with historical experience with rituximab alone. This strategy should be explored further in HCL [90,91].

NEW ANTIGEN TARGETS

The Ig superfamily receptor translocation-associated 2 (IRTA2) gene has been identified in several B-cell malignancies as Fc receptor homolog 5 [92]. Five IRTA family members have been identified, with genes coding for novel members of the Ig receptor family [93]. Cytoplastic domains contain immunoreceptor tyrosine kinase–based activation motifs or immunoreceptor tyrosine-based inhibitory motifs, which suggests a role in cell differentiation and immune responses. Several NHL and HCL cell lines were studied with MoAb's that were developed with specific reactivity to IRTA2 [94]. IRTA2 expression was detected on all cases of HCL assayed, whereas no expression was detected in normal donors. These findings suggest that IRTA2 may be a useful target for future antigen-directed immunotherapy.

SUMMARY

The use of MoAb therapy for the treatment of HCL offers great promise and potential for improving progression-free survival. Rituximab has activity in the setting of previously treated HCL and the ability to eradicate MRD after 2-CdA given as frontline therapy. Alemtuzumab, epratuzumab, Hu-Max-CD20, and other candidate MoAb's should be studied in HCL. Appropriate pharmacologic investigations, use of antigen modulation, and assessments of soluble antigen levels should be considered with future clinical trials of MoAb's in HCL to optimize therapeutic strategies.

References

[1] Bouroncle BA, Wiseman BK, Doan CA. Leukemic reticuloendotheliosis. Blood 1958;13(7): 609–30.

[2] Burns GF, Cawley JC, Worman CP, et al. Multiple heavy chain isotypes on the surface of the cells of hairy cell leukemia. Blood 1978;52(6):1132–47.

[3] Kluin-Nelemans HC, Krouwels MM, Jansen JH, et al. Hairy cell leukemia preferentially expresses the IgG3-subclass. Blood 1990;75(4):972–5.

[4] Forconi F, Sahota SS, Raspadori D, et al. Tumor cells of hairy cell leukemia express multiple clonally related immunoglobulin isotypes via RNA splicing. Blood 2001;98(4):1174–81.

[5] Forconi F, Sahota SS, Raspadori D, et al. Hairy cell leukemia: at the crossroad of somatic mutation and isotype switch. Blood 2004;104(10):3312–7.

[6] Vanhentenrijk V, Tierens A, Wlodarska I, et al. V(H) gene analysis of hairy cell leukemia reveals a homogeneous mutation status and suggests its marginal zone B-cell origin. Leukemia 2004;18(10):1729–32.

[7] Basso K, Liso A, Tiacci E, et al. Gene expression profiling of hairy cell leukemia reveals a phenotype related to memory B cells with altered expression of chemokine and adhesion receptors. J Exp Med 2004;199(1):59–68.

[8] Robbins BA, Ellison DJ, Spinosa JC, et al. Diagnostic application of two-color flow cytometry in 161 cases of hairy cell leukemia. Blood 1993;82(4):1277–87.

[9] Ginaldi L, De Martinis M, Matutes E, et al. Levels of expression of CD19 and CD20 in chronic B cell leukaemias. J Clin Pathol 1998;51(5):364–9.

[10] Quigley MM, Bethel KJ, Sharpe RW, et al. CD52 expression in hairy cell leukemia. Am J Hematol 2003;74(4):227–30.

[11] Sausville JE, Salloum RG, Sorbara L, et al. Minimal residual disease detection in hairy cell leukemia. Comparison of flow cytometric immunophenotyping with clonal analysis using consensus primer polymerase chain reaction for the heavy chain gene. Am J Clin Pathol 2003;119(2):213–7.

[12] Piro LD, Carrera CJ, Carson DA, et al. Lasting remissions in hairy-cell leukemia induced by a single infusion of 2-chlorodeoxyadenosine. N Engl J Med 1990;322(16): 1117–21.

[13] Estey EH, Kurzrock R, Kantarjian HM, et al. Treatment of hairy cell leukemia with 2-chloro-deoxyadenosine (2-CdA). Blood 1992;79(4):882–7.

[14] Piro LD, Ellison DJ, Saven A. The Scripps Clinic experience with 2-chlorodeoxyadenosine in the treatment of hairy cell leukemia. Leuk Lymphoma 1994;14(Suppl 1):121–5.

[15] Tallman MS, Hakimian D, Rademaker AW, et al. Relapse of hairy cell leukemia after 2-chlor-odeoxyadenosine: long-term follow-up of the Northwestern University experience. Blood 1996;88(6):1954–9.

[16] Hoffman MA, Janson D, Rose E, et al. Treatment of hairy-cell leukemia with cladribine: response, toxicity, and long-term follow-up. J Clin Oncol 1997;15(3):1138–42.

[17] Tallman MS, Zakarija A. Hairy cell leukemia: survival and relapse. Long-term follow-up of purine analog-based therapy and approach for relapsed disease. Transfus Apher Sci 2005;32(1):99–103.

[18] Chadha P, Rademaker AW, Mendiratta P, et al. Treatment of hairy cell leukemia with 2-chlor-odeoxyadenosine (2-CdA): long-term follow-up of the Northwestern University experience. Blood 2005;106(1):241–6.

[19] Zinzani PL, Tani M, Marchi E, et al. Long-term follow-up of front-line treatment of hairy cell leukemia with 2-chlorodeoxyadenosine. Haematologica 2004;89(3):309–13.

[20] Jehn U, Bartl R, Dietzfelbinger H, et al. An update: 12-year follow-up of patients with hairy cell leukemia following treatment with 2-chlorodeoxyadenosine. Leukemia 2004;18(9): 1476–81.

[21] Goodman GR, Burian C, Koziol JA, et al. Extended follow-up of patients with hairy cell leukemia after treatment with cladribine. J Clin Oncol 2003;21(5):891–6.

[22] Jansen J, Hermans J. Splenectomy in hairy cell leukemia: a retrospective multicenter analysis. Cancer 1981;47(8):2066–76.

[23] Quesada JR, Reuben J, Manning JT, et al. Alpha interferon for induction of remission in hairy-cell leukemia. N Engl J Med 1984;310(1):15–8.

[24] Worman CP, Catovsky D, Bevan PC, et al. Interferon is effective in hairy-cell leukaemia. Br J Haematol 1985;60(4):759–63.

[25] Ratain MJ, Golomb HM, Vardiman JW, et al. Treatment of hairy cell leukemia with recombinant alpha 2 interferon. Blood 1985;65(3):644–8.

[26] Lauria F, Benfenati D, Raspadori D, et al. Retreatment with 2-CdA of progressed HCL patients. Leuk Lymphoma 1994;14(Suppl 1):143–5.

[27] Kreitman RJ, Wilson WH, Bergeron K, et al. Efficacy of the anti-CD22 recombinant immunotoxin BL22 in chemotherapy-resistant hairy-cell leukemia. N Engl J Med 2001;345(4): 241–7.

[28] Kreitman RJ, Squires DR, Stetler-Stevenson M, et al. Phase I trial of recombinant immunotoxin RFB4(dsFv)-PE38 (BL22) in patients with B-cell malignancies. J Clin Oncol 2005;23(27): 6719–29.

[29] Saven A, Burian C, Koziol JA, et al. Long-term follow-up of patients with hairy cell leukemia after cladribine treatment. Blood 1998;92(6):1918–26.

[30] Seymour JF, Kurzrock R, Freireich EJ, et al. 2-Chlorodeoxyadenosine induces durable remissions and prolonged suppression of $CD4^+$ lymphocyte counts in patients with hairy cell leukemia. Blood 1994;83(10):2906–11.

[31] Betticher DC, Fey MF, von Rohr A, et al. High incidence of infections after 2-chlorodeoxya-denosine (2-CDA) therapy in patients with malignant lymphomas and chronic and acute leu-kaemias. Ann Oncol 1994;5(1):57–64.

[32] Cheson BD. Infectious and immunosuppressive complications of purine analog therapy. J Clin Oncol 1995;13(9):2431–48.

[33] Legrand O, Vekhoff A, Marie JP, et al. Treatment of hairy cell leukaemia (HCL) with 2-chlor-odeoxyadenosine (2-CdA): identification of parameters predictive of adverse effects. Br J Haematol 1997;99(1):165–7.

[34] Ravandi F, O'Brien S. Infections associated with purine analogs and monoclonal anti-bodies. Blood Rev 2005;19(5):253–73.

[35] Albitar M, Do KA, Johnson MM, et al. Free circulating soluble CD52 as a tumor marker in chronic lymphocytic leukemia and its implication in therapy with anti-CD52 antibodies. Cancer 2004;101(5):999–1008.

[36] Lim SH, Davey G, Marcus R. Differential response in a patient treated with Campath-1H monoclonal antibody for refractory non-Hodgkin lymphoma. Lancet 1993;341(8842): 432–3.

[37] Keating MJ, Flinn I, Jain V, et al. Therapeutic role of alemtuzumab (Campath-1H) in patients who have failed fludarabine: results of a large international study. Blood 2002;99(10): 3554–61.

[38] Coleman M, Goldenberg DM, Siegel AB, et al. Epratuzumab: targeting B-cell malignancies through CD22. Clin Cancer Res 2003;9(10 Pt 2):3991S–4S.

[39] Anderson KC, Bates MP, Slaughenhoupt BL, et al. Expression of human B cell-associated an-tigens on leukemias and lymphomas: a model of human B cell differentiation. Blood 1984;63(6):1424–33.

[40] Einfeld DA, Brown JP, Valentine MA, et al. Molecular cloning of the human B cell CD20 re-ceptor predicts a hydrophobic protein with multiple transmembrane domains. EMBO J 1988;7(3):711–7.

[41] Valentine MA, Meier KE, Rossie S, et al. Phosphorylation of the CD20 phosphoprotein in rest-ing B lymphocytes. Regulation by protein kinase C. J Biol Chem 1989;264(19):11282–7.

[42] Tedder TF, Boyd AW, Freedman AS, et al. The B cell surface molecule B1 is functionally linked with B cell activation and differentiation. J Immunol 1985;135(2):973–9.

[43] Reff ME, Carner K, Chambers KS, et al. Depletion of B cells in vivo by a chimeric mouse human monoclonal antibody to CD20. Blood 1994;83(2):435–45.

[44] Maloney DG, Grillo-Lopez AJ, White CA, et al. IDEC-C2B8 (Rituximab) anti-CD20 monoclo-nal antibody therapy in patients with relapsed low-grade non-Hodgkin's lymphoma. Blood 1997;90(6):2188–95.

[45] McLaughlin P, Grillo-Lopez AJ, Link BK, et al. Rituximab chimeric anti-CD20 monoclonal antibody therapy for relapsed indolent lymphoma: half of patients respond to a four-dose treatment program. J Clin Oncol 1998;16(8):2825–33.

[46] Piro LD, White CA, Grillo-Lopez AJ, et al. Extended rituximab (anti-CD20 monoclonal anti-body) therapy for relapsed or refractory low-grade or follicular non-Hodgkin's lymphoma. Ann Oncol 1999;10(6):655–61.

[47] O'Brien SM, Kantarjian H, Thomas DA, et al. Rituximab dose-escalation trial in chronic lym-phocytic leukemia. J Clin Oncol 2001;19(8):2165–70.

[48] Byrd JC, Murphy T, Howard RS, et al. Rituximab using a thrice weekly dosing schedule in B-cell chronic lymphocytic leukemia and small lymphocytic lymphoma demonstrates clinical activity and acceptable toxicity. J Clin Oncol 2001;19(8):2153–64.

[49] Manshouri T, Do KA, Wang X, et al. Circulating CD20 is detectable in the plasma of patients with chronic lymphocytic leukemia and is of prognostic significance. Blood 2003;101(7): 2507–13.

[50] Hagberg H, Lundholm L. Rituximab a chimaeric anti-CD20 monoclonal antibody, in the treatment of hairy cell leukaemia. Br J Haematol 2001;115(3):609–11.

[51] Lauria F, Lenoci M, Annino L, et al. Efficacy of anti-CD20 monoclonal antibodies (Mabthera) in patients with progressed hairy cell leukemia. Haematologica 2001;86(10):1046–50.

[52] Nieva J, Bethel K, Saven A. Phase 2 study of rituximab in the treatment of cladribine-failed patients with hairy cell leukemia. Blood 2003;102(3):810–3.

[53] Thomas DA, O'Brien S, Bueso-Ramos C, et al. Rituximab in relapsed or refractory hairy cell leukemia. Blood 2003;102(12):3906–11.

[54] Zinzani PL, Ascani S, Piccaluga PP, et al. Efficacy of rituximab in hairy cell leukemia treatment. J Clin Oncol 2000;18(22):3875–7.

[55] Hoffman M, Auerbach L. Bone marrow remission of hairy cell leukaemia induced by rituximab (anti-CD20 monoclonal antibody) in a patient refractory to cladribine. Br J Haematol 2000;109(4):900–1.

[56] Pollio F, Pocali B, Palmieri S, et al. Rituximab: a useful drug for a repeatedly relapsed hairy cell leukemia patient. Ann Hematol 2002;81(12):736–8.

[57] Weng WK, Levy R. Two immunoglobulin G fragment C receptor polymorphisms independently predict response to rituximab in patients with follicular lymphoma. J Clin Oncol 2003;21(21):3940–7.

[58] Farag SS, Flinn IW, Modali R, et al. Fc gamma RIIIa and Fc gamma RIIa polymorphisms do not predict response to rituximab in B-cell chronic lymphocytic leukemia. Blood 2004;103(4):1472–4.

[59] Teeling JL, French RR, Cragg MS, et al. Characterization of new human CD20 monoclonal antibodies with potent cytolytic activity against non-Hodgkin lymphomas. Blood 2004;104(6):1793–800.

[60] Stein R, Qu Z, Chen S, et al. Characterization of a new humanized anti-CD20 monoclonal antibody, IMMU-106, and its use in combination with the humanized anti-CD22 antibody, epratuzumab, for the therapy of non-Hodgkin's lymphoma. Clin Cancer Res 2004;10(8): 2868–78.

[61] Nagajothi N, Matsui WH, Mukhina GL, et al. Enhanced cytotoxicity of rituximab following genetic and biochemical disruption of glycosylphosphatidylinositol anchored proteins. Leuk Lymphoma 2004;45(4):795–9.

[62] Filleul B, Delannoy A, Ferrant A, et al. A single course of 2-chloro-deoxyadenosine does not eradicate leukemic cells in hairy cell leukemia patients in complete remission. Leukemia 1994;8(7):1153–6.

[63] Wheaton S, Tallman MS, Hakimian D, et al. Minimal residual disease may predict bone marrow relapse in patients with hairy cell leukemia treated with 2-chlorodeoxyadenosine. Blood 1996;87(4):1556–60.

[64] Matutes E, Meeus P, McLennan K, et al. The significance of minimal residual disease in hairy cell leukaemia treated with deoxycoformycin: a long-term follow-up study. Br J Haematol 1997;98(2):375–83.

[65] Di Gaetano N, Xiao Y, Erba E, et al. Synergism between fludarabine and rituximab revealed in a follicular lymphoma cell line resistant to the cytotoxic activity of either drug alone. Br J Haematol 2001;114(4):800–9.

[66] Cervetti G, Galimberti S, Andreazzoli F, et al. Rituximab as treatment for minimal residual disease in hairy cell leukaemia. Eur J Haematol 2004;73(6):412–7.

[67] Ravandi F, Jorgensen JL, O'Brien SM, et al. Eradication of minimal residual disease (MRD) in hairy cell leukemia (HCL). Blood 2006;107(12):4658–62.

[68] Keating MJ, O'Brien S, Albitar M, et al. Early results of a chemoimmunotherapy regimen of fludarabine, cyclophosphamide, and rituximab as initial therapy for chronic lymphocytic leukemia. J Clin Oncol 2005;23(18):4079–88.

[69] Byrd JC, Rai K, Peterson BL, et al. Addition of rituximab to fludarabine may prolong progression-free survival and overall survival in patients with previously untreated chronic lymphocytic leukemia: an updated retrospective comparative analysis of CALGB 9712 and CALGB 9011. Blood 2005;105(1):49–53.

[70] Ginaldi L, De Martinis M, Matutes E, et al. Levels of expression of CD52 in normal and leukemic B and T cells: correlation with in vivo therapeutic responses to Campath-1H. Leuk Res 1998;22(2):185–91.

[71] Faderl S, Coutre S, Byrd JC, et al. The evolving role of alemtuzumab in management of patients with CLL. Leukemia 2005;19(12):2147–52.

[72] Hale G, Swirsky D, Waldmann H, et al. Reactivity of rat monoclonal antibody CAMPATH-1 with human leukaemia cells and its possible application for autologous bone marrow transplantation. Br J Haematol 1985;60(1):41–8.

[73] Hale G, Xia MQ, Tighe HP, et al. The CAMPATH-1 antigen (CDw52). Tissue Antigens 1990;35(3):118–27.

[74] Dyer MJ. The role of CAMPATH-1 antibodies in the treatment of lymphoid malignancies. Semin Oncol 1999;26(5) (Suppl 14):52–7.

[75] Belov L, de la Vega O, dos Remedios CG, et al. Immunophenotyping of leukemias using a cluster of differentiation antibody microarray. Cancer Res 2001;61(11):4483–9.

[76] Fietz T, Rieger K, Schmittel A, et al. Alemtuzumab (Campath 1H) in hairy cell leukaemia relapsing after rituximab treatment. Hematol J 2004;5(5):451–2.

[77] Cordone I, Annino L, Masi S, et al. Diagnostic relevance of peripheral blood immunocytochemistry in hairy cell leukaemia. J Clin Pathol 1995;48(10):955–60.

[78] Engel P, Nojima Y, Rothstein D, et al. The same epitope on CD22 of B lymphocytes mediates the adhesion of erythrocytes, T and B lymphocytes, neutrophils, and monocytes. J Immunol 1993;150(11):4719–32.

[79] Engel P. CD22. J Biol Regul Homeost Agents 2000;14(4):295–8.

[80] Siegel AB, Goldenberg DM, Cesano A, et al. CD22-directed monoclonal antibody therapy for lymphoma. Semin Oncol 2003;30(4):457–64.

[81] Carnahan J, Wang P, Kendall R, et al. Epratuzumab, a humanized monoclonal antibody targeting CD22: characterization of in vitro properties. Clin Cancer Res 2003;9(10 Pt 2): 3982S–90S.

[82] Shih LB, Lu HH, Xuan H, et al. Internalization and intracellular processing of an anti-B-cell lymphoma monoclonal antibody, LL2. Int J Cancer 1994;56(4):538–45.

[83] Leonard JP, Coleman M, Ketas JC, et al. Phase I/II trial of epratuzumab (humanized anti-CD22 antibody) in indolent non-Hodgkin's lymphoma. J Clin Oncol 2003;21(16):3051–9.

[84] Leonard JP, Coleman M, Ketas JC, et al. Epratuzumab, a humanized anti-CD22 antibody, in aggressive non-Hodgkin's lymphoma: phase I/II clinical trial results. Clin Cancer Res 2004;10(16):5327–34.

[85] Faderl S, Thomas DA, O'Brien S, et al. Experience with alemtuzumab plus rituximab in 2 patients with relapsed and refractory lymphoid malignancies. Blood 2003;101(9): 3413–5.

[86] Leonard JP, Coleman M, Ketas J, et al. Combination antibody therapy with epratuzumab and rituximab in relapsed or refractory non-Hodgkin's lymphoma. J Clin Oncol 2005; 23(22):5044–51.

[87] Venugopal P, Sivaraman S, Huang XK, et al. Effects of cytokines on CD20 antigen expression on tumor cells from patients with chronic lymphocytic leukemia. Leuk Res 2000;24(5): 411–5.

[88] Stockmeyer B, Elsasser D, Dechant M, et al. Mechanisms of G-CSF- or GM-CSF-stimulated tumor cell killing by Fc receptor-directed bispecific antibodies. J Immunol Methods 2001;248(1–2):103–11.

[89] Hernandez-Ilizaliturri FJ, Jupudy V, Reising S, et al. Concurrent administration of granulocyte colony-stimulating factor or granulocyte-monocyte colony-stimulating factor enhances the biological activity of rituximab in a severe combined immunodeficiency mouse lymphoma model. Leuk Lymphoma 2005;46(12):1775–84.

[90] Ferrajoli A, O'Brien SM, Faderl SH, et al. Rituximab plus GM-CSF for patients with chronic lymphocytic leukemia. Blood 2005;106(Suppl 1):214a.

[91] Rossi JF, Lu ZY, Quittet P, et al. Rituximab activity is potentiated by GM-CSF in patients with relapsed, follicular lymphoma: results of a phase II study. Blood 2005;106(Suppl 1):684a.

[92] Davis RS, Wang YH, Kubagawa H, et al. Identification of a family of Fc receptor homologs with preferential B cell expression. Proc Natl Acad Sci U S A 2001;98(17):9772–7.

[93] Davis RS, Dennis G Jr, Kubagawa H, et al. Fc receptor homologs (FcRH1–5) extend the Fc receptor family. Curr Top Microbiol Immunol 2002;266:85–112.

[94] Ise T, Maeda H, Santora K, et al. Immunoglobulin superfamily receptor translocation associated 2 protein on lymphoma cell lines and hairy cell leukemia cells detected by novel monoclonal antibodies. Clin Cancer Res 2005;11(1):87–96.

Hematol Oncol Clin N Am 20 (2006) 1137–1151

HEMATOLOGY/ONCOLOGY CLINICS
OF NORTH AMERICA

SEVIER
UNDERS

Immunotoxins in the Treatment of Refractory Hairy Cell Leukemia

Robert J. Kreitman, MD[a],*, Ira Pastan, MD[b]

[a]Clinical Immunotherapy Section, Laboratory of Molecular Biology,
Center for Cancer Research, National Cancer Institute, National Institutes of Health,
9000 Rockville Pike, Building 37, Room 5124b, Bethesda, MD 20892-4255, USA
[b]Laboratory of Molecular Biology, Center for Cancer Research,
National Cancer Institute, National Institutes of Health, 9000 Rockville Pike,
Building 37, Room 5106, Bethesda, MD 20892-4255, USA

REFRACTORY HAIRY CELL LEUKEMIA

As detailed elsewhere in this issue, hairy cell leukemia (HCL) is one of the most treatable disorders, with long-term (>5 year) complete remissions (CRs) possible in most patients who are treated with purine analogs cladribine and pentostatin. Recent studies showed response rates of 95% to 100% with either agent. CR rates are 79% to 95%, and most patients remain in CR at median follow-up times of 9 to 15 years [1–3]. Moreover, 50% to 70% of patients who undergo a second course of cladribine achieve CR [1,2,4]. Despite these excellent results, refractory HCL is a problem with increasing clinical importance. This is based on the absence of a plateau in the disease-free survival curves for patients who are treated with pentostatin or cladribine [1,2,4], which indicates that these agents are not curative. Polymerase chain reaction and Southern blot analyses of patients in CR after cladribine also confirm lack of cure [5,6]. Second or later courses of purine analogs are associated with lower CR rates and decreased response durability. Thus, with enough time since the introduction of purine analogs for this disease, one would expect an accumulation of patients who have purine analog refractory HCL, particularly those who are young or who do not die of other causes.

RATIONALE FOR SURFACE-TARGETED THERAPY FOR HAIRY CELL LEUKEMIA

Although HCL becomes refractory to purine analog therapy, the HCL cells do not change their immunophenotypic characteristics (see the article by Sharpe & Bethel elsewhere in this issue). Thus, many of the surface molecules that are expressed at high levels by HCL, particularly CD20, CD22, CD25, and

---

*Corresponding author. E-mail address: kreitmar@mail.nih.gov (R.J. Kreitman).

0889-8588/06/$ – see front matter
doi:10.1016/j.hoc.2006.06.009

Published by Elsevier Inc.
hemonc.theclinics.com

CD11c, constitute potential targets for monoclonal antibody (Mab)-directed therapy. HCL is an ideal disease for targeting antibodies, because HCL cells generally are not packed tightly in the bone marrow, lymph nodes are uncommon except after splenectomy, and HCL cells in the spleen and blood are accessible to protein that is injected into the bloodstream. Moreover, approaches that use biologic therapy avoid the cumulative myelosuppressive and immunosuppressive effects of repeated courses of purine analog, which can decrease $CD4^+$ T-cell numbers for up to 4 years [7,8].

MECHANISM OF CYTOTOXICITY OF PROTEIN TOXINS

Protein toxins include bacterial and plant toxins. They are effective cell-killing agents because they inhibit protein synthesis catalytically; several are capable of killing a cell when only one molecule is placed into the cytoplasm [9,10]. Plant toxins include ricin, abrin, mistletoe lectin, modeccin, pokeweed antiviral protein, saporin, Bryodin 1, bouganin, and gelonin [11]. Bacterial toxins include Shiga toxin, *Escherichia coli*–derived Shiga-like toxin, anthrax toxin, diphtheria toxin (DT), and *Pseudomonas* exotoxin (PE) [12,13]. Of all of these toxins, only PE and DT exist in single-chain forms that contain binding and activity domains. Hence, PE and DT are easiest to convert into single-chain cancer cell–specific toxins by replacing the binding domain with a specific ligand for tumor cells. Both PE and DT work catalytically ADP ribosylating elongation factor-2 in the cytosol [14–16]. PE was used to target HCL; the public is not immunized against this toxin.

MECHANISM OF INTOXICATION OF *PSEUDOMONAS* EXOTOXIN

The full-length 613–amino acid PE molecule contains three functional domains [17,18], including domain Ia (amino acids 1–252) for cell binding, domain II (amino acids 253–364) for translocating the toxin to the cytosol, and domain III (amino acids 400–613) for ADP ribosylating and inactivating elongation factor-2 in the cytosol. Domain Ib (amino acids 365–399) connects domains II and III. These three steps of intoxication are shown in Fig. 1 for the molecule BL22. To target PE to cells without binding to normal cells, domain Ia is removed, and nonessential amino acids, including a disulfide bond, also are removed, which leaves a 38-kd fragment (amino acids 253–364 and 381–613) that is called PE38 [19,20]. The ligand is conjugated chemically to PE38 or fused to the amino terminus of the toxin. Fusion toxins have several potential advantages over chemical conjugates, including smaller size and increased ability to exit the bloodstream, ease of production, a defined toxin–ligand junction, and the ability to create mutants to improve activity. Instead of targeting using a Mab, an Fv fragment of a Mab is used. As shown in Fig. 2, the Fv fragment may be single chain, containing a peptide linker between the variable heavy (VH) and light (VL) domains [21–23]. Alternatively, the Fv may be stabilized by a disulfide bond by mutating V_H and V_L residues to cysteine [24,25]. In

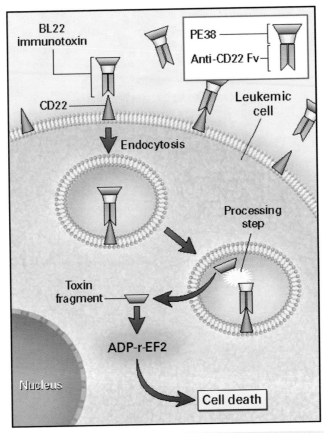

Fig. 1. Intoxication of cells by BL22. BL22 binds to CD22, enters by endocytosis, is processed and translocated to the cytosol where it ADP-ribosylates elongation factor 2 (EF2) and causes death of the leukemia cell. (*From* Kreitman RJ, Wilson WH, Bergeron K, et al. Efficacy of the anti-CD22 recombinant immunotoxin BL22 in chemotherapy-resistant hairy-cell leukemia. N Engl J Med 2001;345:242; with permission.)

either case, one of the variable domains is fused to the amino terminus of PE38, which results in a recombinant immunotoxin.

ANTI-CD25 RECOMBINANT IMMUNOTOXIN LMB-2 AGAINST HAIRY CELL LEUKEMIA

Rationale and Preclinical Development of LMB-2

The interleukin (IL)-2 receptor (IL2R) is composed of α (CD25), β (CD122), and γ (CD132) chains. IL-2 binds with high affinity (kd~10^{-11} M) to the complex of all three, but with low affinity (kd~10^{-8} M) to CD25 alone [26]. In malignant tumors that express IL2R, including HCL, CD25 is expressed most commonly, often in the absence of other IL2R segments [27–29]. To

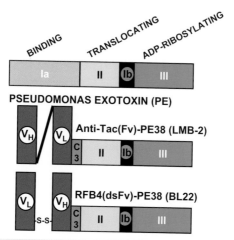

Fig. 2. Structure of PE and recombinant immunotoxins.

target CD25 on cells, the high-affinity Mab anti-Tac was used [30]. The recombinant immunotoxin LMB-2 contains the variable domains of anti-Tac connected by way of a peptide linker, and VH is fused to PE38. LMB-2 resulted in complete regressions of CD25+ human xenografts in mice [31,32], and killed fresh leukemic cells from patients who had a variety of T- and B-cell leukemias [20,32–34]. Primary HCL cells were particularly sensitive, with IC50s (concentration required for 50% inhibition) of 0.5 to 6 ng/mL on cells that expressed 1250 to 7200 sites/cell of CD25 [34].

Phase I Results of LMB-2

LMB-2 was administered to 35 patients who had chemotherapy-resistant leukemia, lymphoma, and Hodgkin's disease [35]. The maximum tolerated dosage (MTD) was 40 µg/kg every other day for three days (QOD × 3). As shown in Fig. 3A, the most common nondose-limiting toxicities at 30 to 50 µg/kg QOD × 3 were transaminase elevations, hypoalbuminemia, fever, nausea, fatigue, and edema. Immunogenicity from LMB-2 was infrequent, with 6 out of 35 patients unable to receive further treatment because of neutralizing antibodies developing after cycle one [35]. The median half-life of LMB-2 at the MTD was about 4 hours. Four of the 35 patients had HCL (Table 1). All 4 of these patients had experienced failure of at least cladribine and interferon, and yet all had major responses to LMB-2 [36]. Before treatment, Patient L230 (Fig. 4A) had transfusion dependence for red blood cells, and had a platelet count of 47,000/mm³, absolute neutrophil count (ANC) of 360/mm³, and had enlargement in spleen and precarinal lymph nodes. The hairy cell count was 478/mm³ and decreased by more than 90% after just one dosage of LMB-2, as assessed on day 3 before the second dosage. By day 8, HCL cells had decreased by more than 99% to 3.0/mm³, and were cleared completely

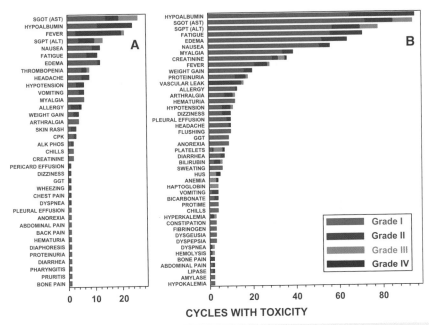

Fig. 3. Toxicity of BL22. LMB-2– (A) and BL22–related (B) adverse events in patients who were treated at dosage levels of 30 to 50 µg/kg QOD × 3. Included are 30 cycles of LMB-2 in 20 patients (A) and 172 cycles of BL22 in 34 patients (B). ALK PHOS, alkaline phosphate; ALT, alanine aminotransferase; AST, aspartate aminotransferase; CPK, creatinine phosphokinase; GGT, gamma glutamyl transferase; HUS, hemolytic uremic syndrome; PROTIME, prothrombin time; SGOT, serum glutamic-oxaloacetic transaminase; SGPT, serum glutamic-pyruvic transaminase. (*From* Kreitman RJ, Squires DR, Stetler-Stevenson M, et al. Phase I trial of recombinant immunotoxin RFB4(dsFv)-PE38 (BL22) in patients with B-cell malignancies. J Clin Oncol 2005;23:6724; with permission.)

following cycle 2. Flow cytometry is sensitive to about 0.01% to 0.005%. CR in Patient L230 included resolution of splenomegaly and precarinal adenopathy, transfusion independence, and reversal of cytopenias (see Fig. 3A). The platelet count was the first to recover, followed by improvement in granulocyte count. The hemoglobin improved to greater than 11 g/dL later (by 150 days) and remained above that level for 7.5 years without further treatment. During that time, the platelets stayed greater than 100,000/mm^3, but the ANC decreased gradually to 500/mm^3. This patient has just enrolled in the phase II trial of BL22 (see later discussion), and has achieved CR with one cycle of BL22. The other 3 patients who had HCL and were treated with LMB-2 had partial response (PR) after one cycle of 30, 63, and 40 µg/kg QOD × 3, with greater than 98% to 99.8% decreases in circulating HCL cells. CR was not achieved in these patients, probably because they could not be retreated effectively because of infections, dose limiting toxicity (DLT), or neutralizing antibodies.

Table 1
Clinical characteristics of LMB-2 and BL22

Clinical data	LMB-2	BL22
Target	CD25	CD22
Patients with HCL cells positive for target	80%	100%
Total patients treated on phase I	35	46
Cycle 1 MTD (µg/kg QOD × 3)	40	40
Patients who have HCL only:		
Total patients treated in phase I	4	31
Patients who have HCLv	0	3
Median age (range)	63 (48–66)	54 (30–81)
Men-Women	3–1	25–6
Median (range) previous courses cladribine	4 (1–5)	2 (1–7)
Previous courses pentostatin	0–1	0–3
CRs to immunotoxin	1 of 4 (25%)	19 of 31 (61%)
PRs to immunotoxin	3 of 4 (75%)	6 of 31 (19%)
Response rate	100%	81%
Hematologic remission[a]	1 of 4 (25%)	22 of 30 (73%)
Immunogenicity	1 of 4 (25%)	11 of 31 (35%)
Median half-life at 30–50 µg/kg IV	250 min	180 min

Abbreviations: IV, intravenous; HCLV, HCL variant.

[a]Hematologic remission defined as ANC, platelets, and hemoglobin at least 1500/mm^3, 100,000/mm^3 and 11 g/dL, respectively.

Data from Refs. [35,36,49,50].

ANTI-CD22 RECOMBINANT IMMUNOTOXIN BL22 AGAINST HAIRY CELL LEUKEMIA

Rationale and Preclinical Development of BL22

Before the development of BL22, several chemical conjugates that contain plant toxins were constructed to target CD22 on B-cell malignancies [37–42]. PE originally was targeted to CD22 using the MAb LL2, which resulted in complete regression in preclinical xenograft models [43,44]. LL2 was not stable enough as a single chain Fv to make a recombinant immunotoxin, however. RFB4 was stable as a single chain or as a disulfide-stabilized Fv, which allowed the production of recombinant anti-CD22 immunotoxins [45,46]. BL22 contained a disulfide bond between cysteine residues replacing framework residues Arg44 of V_H and Gly100 of V_L. The disulfide-stabilized immunotoxin (see Fig. 2), termed RFB4(dsFv)-PE38 or BL22, is fully recombinant because the disulfide bond between V_L and V_H-PE38 forms naturally during in vitro renaturation of the two fragments, and chemical conjugation is not needed. Complete regressions in

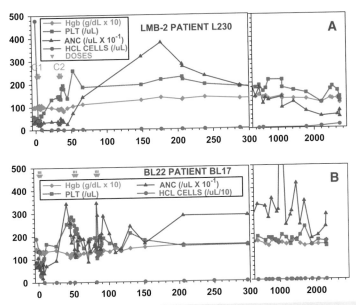

Fig. 4. Complete remission of patients who have HCL to recombinant immunotoxins. LMB-2 Patient L230 (A) received two cycles of LMB-2 at 63 µg/kg QOD × 3. The three dosages of each cycle are indicated by a coalescence of three arrows. The hemoglobin (Hgb), platelet count (PLT), absolute neutrophil count (ANC), and circulating HCL count (HCL) are shown from several days before to 300 days after the first dosage, and is followed by graphs showing counts during the following 5 to 6 years. Similar data are shown for BL22 patient BL17 (B) who received three cycles of BL22 at 30 µg/kg QOD × 3.

mice of human $CD22^+$ B-cell lymphoma xenografts were observed with BL22 at plasma levels that could be tolerated in Cynomolgus monkeys [47]. Leukemic cells freshly obtained from patients also were sensitive ex vivo to BL22 [48].

Clinical Testing of BL22 and Overall Phase I Results

BL22 was administered to 46 patients who had B-cell leukemias and lymphomas [49,50]. Thirty-one 31 had HCL, 4 patients had non-Hodgkin's lymphoma (NHL), and 11 patients had chronic lymphocytic leukemia. A total of 265 cycles was administered to 46 patients at 3 to 50 µg/kg QOD × 3. Serious toxicity included hemolytic uremic syndrome (HUS) observed in 1 patient who had NHL during cycle 1, and in 4 patients who had HCL during retreatment on cycles 2 or 3. The only other DLT was cytokine release syndrome in a patient who had HCL who received cycle 2 of BL22 and had acute fever, hypotension, and bone pain that resolved completely after several days. The MTD for cycle 1 was defined as 40 µg/kg QOD × 3, in that all 12 patients who were enrolled at this dosage level tolerated cycle 1 well without DLT. The most common toxicities of BL22 were fatigue, myalgia, alanine aminotransferase and aspartate aminotransferase elevations, and hypoalbuminemia (see Fig. 3B). Grade 3 transaminase elevations are not considered dose-limiting, because of the absence of evidence of functional hepatic impairment, and grade 3 transaminase elevations resolved in less than 4 days. Weight gain was observed, which probably was due, at least in part, to vascular leak syndrome (VLS), but VLS did not lead to pulmonary edema. Unlike purine analogs in patients who have HCL [7,8], BL22 did not cause decreases in CD4 counts. Neutralizing antibodies to BL22, as assessed by incubating purified BL22 with patient serum and determining the percentage loss of cytotoxicity toward a CD22-expressing cell line, developed in 11 patients (all HCL) after 1 to 8 cycles of BL22. Plasma levels were determined by incubating plasma dilutions against cell line and comparing cytotoxicity using a standard curve made from purified BL22. Pharmacokinetics showed that peak levels were dosage related and that median half-lives were about 3 hours at 30 to 50 μg/kg QOD × 3. Although plasma levels were dosage related, variability within dosage levels was extensive owing to the high expression of CD22 on HCL cells, which caused a sink effect, particularly at high levels of tumor burden.

Response to BL22 in Patients Who Have Hairy Cell Leukemia in the Phase I Study

As shown in Table 1, patients who had HCL were pretreated significantly, with one to seven previous courses of purine analog, including cladribine and pentostatin; frequently, patients also had undergone splenectomy, interferon, fludarabine, rituximab, and other chemotherapy. Nevertheless, response to BL22 in HCL was high with 19 of 31 patients (61%) achieving CR and 6 patients (19%) achieving PR, for an overall response rate of 81% in this phase I trial. Of 3 patients who were enrolled and had HCL variant, all had CR. Although response did not require resolution of cytopenias, the authors found that all CRs, two of six PRs and 1 patient with a marginal response had resolution of pre-existing cytopenias to at least ANC, platelets, and hemoglobin of 1500/mm^3, 100,000/mm^3, and 11 g/dL, respectively. Similar to the patient who had HCL with CR to LMB-2, patients with CR typically had more than 90% clearance of circulating HCL cells by 2 days (before the second dosage), and 99% clearance by 1 week. Lack of major response was associated with low doses (2 patients) or massive abdominal adenopathy (2 patients). Neutralizing antibodies were observed in 11 of 31 patients who had HCL and in several cases prevented achievement of maximal response; however, 5 CRs and two PRs were achieved in these 11 patients. Of the 19 CRs, 11 were observed after cycle 1 and 8 required 2 to 14 cycles before CR could be documented. The CR rate was dosage-related in that 12 (86%) of the patients who were enrolled at 40 to 50 μg/kg QOD × 3 achieved CR, compared with 7 (41%) of the patients who were enrolled at lower dosages ($P = .011$). Of the 19 CRs, 10 patients (53%) never had achieved CR to previous therapy, 6 patients (19%) had no response to the last course of purine analog, 2 (6%) patients had a CR of less than 6 months to the last course of cladribine, and 1 (3%) patient had a CR of less than 2 years to the last course of cladribine. Thus, patients who had chemoresistant HCL had a high response rate to BL22 in phase I studies, and responses were not influenced by previous lack of response to purine analog.

Duration of Response to BL22 in Patients Who Have Hairy Cell Leukemia

As shown in Fig. 5A, the median duration of CR was 36 months (range, 5–73 months). Seven of the 19 CRs (37%) are still present at a median of 51 months (range, 35–73 months). Resolution of cytopenias, as defined above, which is lifesaving in HCL, was observed in 22 of 30 patients (73%) who had baseline cytopenias (Fig. 5B). The median duration of resolution of cytopenias was 38 months (range, 4–73 months), and 9 of 22 patients (41%) are still in hematologic remission at a median follow-up of 50 months (range, 35–73 months).

Response in Patients Who Have Hairy Cell Leukemia with Different Levels of Tumor Burden

As shown in Fig. 6, patients who had HCL had different levels of tumor burden at the time that they began BL22. A typical patient who has classic HCL, as shown in Fig. 6B, has an enlarged spleen and low numbers of circulating HCL cells. This patient (BL23) had a CR with one cycle and had one consolidation cycle. After splenectomy, patients who have classic HCL can have high levels of circulating cells, as shown in Fig. 6A (BL25). This patient had CR after three cycles and had one consolidation cycle. Patient BL17 had classic HCL, an enlarged spleen, and, as shown in Fig. 4B, had a high number of circulating HCL cells ($1550/mm^3$). This patient had a CR documented after cycle 1, and received 2 consolidation cycles. The ANC was not consistently above $1500/mm^3$ until after cycle 3, but this patient has remained in CR for over 6 years. Patients who have HCL variant typically have high levels of circulating HCL cells, whether they have had splenectomy (Fig. 6D) or not (Fig. 6C). Patient BL14 had CR after nine cycles followed by two consolidation cycles (see Fig. 6C), although patient BL26 had CR after one cycle, followed by two consolidation cycles (see Fig. 6D). Thus, tumor burden does not prevent

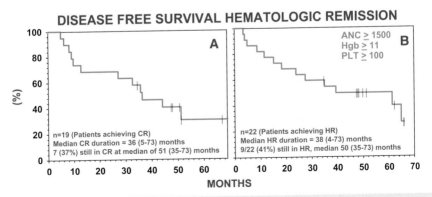

Fig. 5. Duration of response. Disease-free survival curves for CR (A) and hematologic remission (B). Vertical red lines indicate follow-up times for patients remaining in remission.

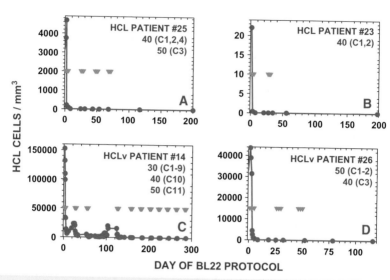

Fig. 6. Eradication of circulating HCL cells. (*A, B*) Classic HCL. (*C, D*) HCL variant. Three overlapping pink triangles indicate three dosages of BL22 per cycle. Dosage levels in µg/kg QOD × 3 (*in blue*). Patient #14 required splenectomy after cycle 3 to resolve HCL-related coagulopathy, followed by progressive disease in the blood and marrow. (*From* Kreitman RJ, Squires DR, Stetler-Stevenson M, et al. Phase I trial of recombinant immunotoxin RFB4(dsFv)-PE38 (BL22) in patients with B-cell malignancies. J Clin Oncol 2005;23:6727; with permission.)

achievement of CR by BL22, but, partly because of the sink effect and partly because of tumor penetration, patients with high tumor burden may require extra cycles for optimal response.

Minimal Residual Disease in Hairy Cell Leukemia After BL22

CR in HCL is defined as absence of HCL in blood, marrow, and lymph nodes by conventional microscopic and radiographic studies, and a decrease in spleen size to normal. CR with minimal residual disease is defined as collections of HCL cells visible by immunohistochemistry for CD20 in the bone marrow biopsy [51], or HCL cells present in the blood by flow cytometry [49,50]. The authors found that minimal residual disease was detected after CR in 1 of 19 patients (5%) by immunohistochemistry, and in 2 patients (11%) by flow cytometry of the blood.

DISCUSSION AND FUTURE PLANS WITH HAIRY CELL LEUKEMIA IMMUNOTOXINS

Targeting Hairy Cell Leukemia with LMB-2 Versus BL22

Although most of the CRs were observed with BL22, few patients who have HCL have received LMB-2, and it is not possible to determine which agent is better for this disease. Clearly, in the 20% of patients that have HCL with CD25-negative HCL cells, BL22 is the better immunotoxin. One of the patients (L235) who received LMB-2 had a minor population of CD25-negative HCL cells that were selected for after response to LMB-2, but all of these HCL cells remained bright positive for CD22. The authors have not observed selection by BL22 of CD22-negative or dim cells. For these reasons, patients who have HCL are undergoing phase II testing with BL22, and LMB-2 is undergoing phase II testing in other diseases, including chronic lymphocytic leukemia and CTCL. It is possible that LMB-2 may be of use in a minority of patients unable to obtain CR with BL22, however. Because only small amounts of BL22 can be given to patients (3–4 mg per dosage), the sink effect of $CD22^+$ cells may be overwhelming for some patients, and this "binding site barrier" as proposed experimentally [52], may prevent adequate distribution of BL22 to all tumor cells. Because patients who have HCL have about one tenth the level of CD25 expression as CD22 expression, some patients who have HCL may achieve better tumor distribution with LMB-2 compared with BL22. Additionally, some patients may be particularly sensitive to HUS with BL22, and may be better candidates for LMB-2, which has not caused HUS. Other treatment options are limited for these patients. For these reasons, phase II testing of LMB-2 in patients who have had previous BL22 therapy has been approved.

Mechanism of Hemolytic Uremic Syndrome in Patients Who Are Treated with BL22

In all five patients who had HUS (1 NHL, 4 HCL), plus a sixth special exemption patient who had HCL, von Willebrand factor-cleaving metalloprotease (ADAMTS-13) function [53] was unimpaired. Thus, the mechanism of HUS in the authors' patients is not due to high levels of circulating unusually long multimers of von Willebrand factor, as has been observed in thrombotic thrombocytopenic purpura. This suggests not only that HUS that is due to BL22 may not require plasma exchange, but also that the HUS may be prevented or alleviated by antiplatelet agents that generally are not successful for classic HUS–thrombocytopenic purpura. Several hundred cycles of other PE38-containing recombinant toxins have been administered to patients without any detectable HUS, which indicates that the mechanism is related, at least in part, to CD22. All five patients who had HCL and HUS experienced hematologic remissions and three had CRs, which suggests that the risk-benefit ratio clearly is favorable, even in patients who have HUS. A major goal of phase II testing of BL22 in HCL is to avoid HUS in patients who respond to BL22.

Ability to Achieve Maximal Response in Hairy Cell Leukemia

HCL cannot be cured by purine analog therapy, and repeated courses of purine analog for resistant patients lack efficacy and lead to cumulative long-term toxicity to $CD4^+$ T cells. In contrast, recombinant immunotoxins are not associated with cumulative toxicity to T cells. Moreover, even normal B cells, which generally are undetectable during initiation of treatment with immunotoxins, increase with achievement of CR. Although HUS has been observed during treatment cycles 2 and 3 of BL22, it never has occurred during later cycles, even up to a total of 31 cycles. This makes it theoretically possible to continue treating with immunotoxin until the optimal response is achieved. Newer, higher sensitivity tests for HCL, including polymerase chain reaction tests that use clonogenic primers, are being developed to detect as few as 1 in a million HCL cells, and to determine if immunotoxins, which work differently than chemotherapy, can eradicate this disease in some patients.

Acknowledgments

This work was supported by the intramural program of the National Cancer Institutes.

Suggested Readings

Chiron MF, Fryling CM, FitzGerald DJ. Cleavage of *Pseudomonas* exotoxin and diphtheria toxin by a furin-like enzyme prepared from beef liver. J Biol Chem 1994;269:18167–76.

Fryling C, Ogata M, FitzGerald D. Characterization of a cellular protease that cleaves *Pseudomonas* exotoxin. Infect Immun 1992;60:497–502.

Hessler JL, Kreitman RJ. An early step in *Pseudomonas* exotoxin action is removal of the terminal lysine residue, which allows binding to the KDEL receptor. Biochemistry 1997;36: 14577–82.

Kounnas MZ, Morris RE, Thompson MR, et al. The α2-macroglobulin receptor/low density lipoprotein receptor-related protein binds and internalizes *Pseudomonas* exotoxin A. J Biol Chem 1992;267:12420–3.

Kreitman RJ, Pastan I. Importance of the glutamate residue of KDEL in increasing the cytotoxicity of *Pseudomonas* exotoxin derivatives and for increased binding to the KDEL receptor. Biochem J 1995;307:29–37.

Ogata M, Fryling CM, Pastan I, et al. Cell-mediated cleavage of *Pseudomonas* exotoxin between Arg^{279} and Gly^{280} generates the enzymatically active fragment which translocates to the cytosol. J Biol Chem 1992;267:25396–401.

Theuer C, Kasturi S, Pastan I. Domain II of *Pseudomonas* exotoxin A arrests the transfer of translocating nascent chains into mammalian microsomes. Biochemistry 1994;33: 5894–900.

Theuer CP, Buchner J, FitzGerald D, et al. The N-terminal region of the 37-kDa translocated fragment of *Pseudomonas* exotoxin A aborts translocation by promoting its own export after microsomal membrane insertion. Proc Natl Acad Sci U S A 1993;90:7774–8.

References

[1] Else M, Ruchlemer R, Osuji N, et al. Long remissions in hairy cell leukemia with purine analogs—a report of 219 patients with a median follow-up of 12.5 years. Cancer 2005; 104:2442–8.

[2] Chadha P, Rademaker AW, Mendiratta P, et al. Treatment of hairy cell leukemia with 2-chlorodeoxyadenosine (2-CdA): long-term follow-up of the Northwestern University experience. Blood 2005;106:241–6.

[3] Goodman GR, Burian C, Koziol JA, et al. Extended follow-up of patients with hairy cell leukemia after treatment with cladribine. J Clin Oncol 2003;21:891–6.

[4] Saven A, Burian C, Koziol JA, et al. Long-term follow-up of patients with hairy cell leukemia after cladribine treatment. Blood 1998;92:1918–26.

[5] Filleul B, Delannoy A, Ferrant A, et al. A single course of 2-chloro-deoxyadenosine does not eradicate leukemic cells in hairy cell leukemia patients in complete remission. Leukemia 1994;8:1153–6.

[6] Carbone A, Reato G, Di Celle PF, et al. Disease eradication in hairy cell leukemia patients treated with 2-chlorodeoxyadenosine [letter]. Leukemia 1994;8:2019–20.

[7] Seymour JF, Kurzrock R, Freireich EJ, et al. 2-chlorodeoxyadenosine induces durable remissions and prolonged suppression of CD4+ lymphocyte counts in patients with hairy cell leukemia. Blood 1994;83:2906–11.

[8] Seymour JF, Talpaz M, Kurzrock R. Response duration and recovery of CD4+ lymphocytes following deoxycoformycin in interferon-alpha-resistant hairy cell leukemia: 7-year follow-up. Leukemia 1997;11:42–7.

[9] Yamaizumi M, Mekada E, Uchida T, et al. One molecule of diphtheria toxin fragment A introduced into a cell can kill the cell. Cell 1978;15:245–50.

[10] Endo Y, Mitsui K, Motizuki M, et al. The mechanism of action of ricin and related toxic lectins on eukaryotic ribosomes. J Biol Chem 1987;262:5908–12.

[11] Bolognesi A, Polito L, Tazzari PL, et al. In vitro anti-tumour activity of anti-CD80 and anti-CD86 immunotoxins containing type 1 ribosome-inactivating proteins. Br J Haematol 2000;110:351–61.

[12] Moake JL. Thrombotic thrombocytopenic purpura and the hemolytic uremic syndrome. Arch Pathol Lab Med 2002;126:1430–3.

[13] Scobie HM, Young JAT. Interactions between anthrax toxin receptors and protective antigen. Curr Opin Microbiol 2005;8:106–12.

[14] Carroll SF, Collier RJ. Active site of *Pseudomonas aeruginosa* exotoxin A. Glutamic acid 553 is photolabeled by NAD and shows functional homology with glutamic acid 148 of diphtheria toxin. J Biol Chem 1987;262:8707–11.

[15] Uchida T, Pappenheimer AM Jr, Harper AA. Reconstitution of diphtheria toxin from two nontoxic cross-reacting mutant proteins. Science 1972;175:901–3.

[16] Uchida T, Pappenheimer AM Jr, Greany R. Diphtheria toxin and related proteins I. Isolation and properties of mutant proteins serologically related to diphtheria toxin. J Biol Chem 1973;248:3838–44.

[17] Hwang J, FitzGerald DJ, Adhya S, et al. Functional domains of Pseudomonas exotoxin identified by deletion analysis of the gene expressed in *E. coli*. Cell 1987;48:129–36.

[18] Allured VS, Collier RJ, Carroll SF, et al. Structure of exotoxin A of *Pseudomonas aeruginosa* at 3.0 Angstrom resolution. Proc Natl Acad Sci U S A 1986;83:1320–4.

[19] Siegall CB, Chaudhary VK, FitzGerald DJ, et al. Functional analysis of domains II, Ib, and III of *Pseudomonas* exotoxin. J Biol Chem 1989;264:14256–61.

[20] Kreitman RJ, Batra JK, Seetharam S, et al. Single-chain immunotoxin fusions between anti-Tac and *Pseudomonas* exotoxin: relative importance of the two toxin disulfide bonds. Bioconjug Chem 1993;4:112–20.

[21] Chaudhary VK, Queen C, Junghans RP, et al. A recombinant immunotoxin consisting of two antibody variable domains fused to *Pseudomonas* exotoxin. Nature 1989;339:394–7.

[22] Huston JS, Levinson D, Mudgett-Hunter M, et al. Protein engineering of antibody binding sites: recovery of specific activity in an antidigoxin single-chain Fv analogue produced in *Escherichia coli*. Proc Natl Acad Sci U S A 1988;85:5879–83.

[23] Bird RE, Hardman KD, Jacobson JW, et al. Single-chain antigen-binding proteins. Science 1988;242:423–6.

[24] Reiter Y, Brinkmann U, Kreitman RJ, et al. Stabilization of the Fv fragments in recombinant immunotoxins by disulfide bonds engineered into conserved framework regions. Biochemistry 1994;33:5451–9.

[25] Reiter Y, Kreitman RJ, Brinkmann U, et al. Cytotoxic and antitumor activity of a recombinant immunotoxin composed of disulfide-stablized anti-Tac Fv fragment and truncated *Pseudomonas* exotoxin. Int J Cancer 1994;58:142–9.

[26] Taniguchi T, Minami Y. The IL2/IL-2 receptor system: a current overview. Cell 1993;73:5–8.

[27] Kodaka T, Uchiyama T, Ishikawa T, et al. Interleukin-2 receptor β-chain (p70–75) expressed on leukemic cells from adult T cell leukemia patients. Jpn J Cancer Res 1990;81:902–8.

[28] Yagura H, Tamaki T, Furitsu T, et al. Demonstration of high-affinity interleukin-2 receptors on B-chronic lymphocytic leukemia cells: functional and structural characterization. Blut 1990;60:181–6.

[29] Sheibani K, Winberg CD, Velde SVD, et al. Distribution of lymphocytes with interleukin-2 receptors (TAC antigens) in reactive lymphoproliferative processes, Hodgkin's disease, and non-Hodgkin's lymphomas: an immunohistologic study of 300 cases. Am J Pathol 1987;127:27–37.

[30] Uchiyama T, Nelson DL, Fleisher TA, et al. A monoclonal antibody (anti-Tac) reactive with activated and functionally mature human T cells. II. Expression of Tac antigen on activated cytotoxic killer T cells, suppressor cells, and on one of two types of helper T cells. J Immunol 1981;126:1398–403.

[31] Kreitman RJ, Bailon P, Chaudhary VK, et al. Recombinant immunotoxins containing anti-Tac(Fv) and derivatives of Pseudomonas exotoxin produce complete regression in mice of an interleukin-2 receptor-expressing human carcinoma. Blood 1994;83:426–34.

[32] Kreitman RJ, Pastan I. Targeting Pseudomonas exotoxin to hematologic malignancies. Semin Cancer Biol 1995;6:297–306.

[33] Kreitman RJ, Chaudhary VK, Waldmann TA, et al. Cytotoxic activities of recombinant immunotoxins composed of Pseudomonas toxin or diphtheria toxin toward lymphocytes from patients with adult T-cell leukemia. Leukemia 1993;7:553–62.

[34] Robbins DH, Margulies I, Stetler-Stevenson M, et al. Hairy cell leukemia, a B-cell neoplasm which is particularly sensitive to the cytotoxic effect of anti-Tac(Fv)-PE38 (LMB-2). Clin Cancer Res 2000;6:693–700.

[35] Kreitman RJ, Wilson WH, White JD, et al. Phase I trial of recombinant immunotoxin anti-Tac(Fv)-PE38 (LMB-2) in patients with hematologic malignancies. J Clin Oncol 2000;18:1614–36.

[36] Kreitman RJ, Wilson WH, Robbins D, et al. Responses in refractory hairy cell leukemia to a recombinant immunotoxin. Blood 1999;94:3340–8.

[37] Ghetie M-A, May RD, Till M, et al. Evaluation of ricin A chain-containing immunotoxins directed against CD19 and CD22 antigens on normal and malignant human B-cells as potential reagents for in vivo therapy. Cancer Res 1988;48:2610–7.

[38] Ghetie M-A, Richardson J, Tucker T, et al. Antitumor activity of Fab' and IgG-anti-CD22 immunotoxins in disseminated human B lymphoma grown in mice with severe combined immunodeficiency disease: effect on tumor cells in extranodal sites. Cancer Res 1991;51:5876–80.

[39] Bregni M, Siena S, Formosa A, et al. B-cell restricted saporin immunotoxins: activity against B-cell lines and chronic lymphocytic leukemia cells. Blood 1989;73:753–62.

[40] Amlot PL, Stone MJ, Cunningham D, et al. A phase I study of an anti-CD22-deglycosylated ricin A chain immunotoxin in the treatment of B-cell lymphomas resistant to conventional therapy. Blood 1993;82:2624–33.

[41] Sausville EA, Headlee D, Stetler-Stevenson M, et al. Continuous infusion of the anti-CD22 immunotoxin IgG-RFB4-SMPT-dgA in patients with B-cell lymphoma: a phase I study. Blood 1995;85:3457–65.

[42] Senderowicz AM, Vitetta E, Headlee D, et al. Complete sustained response of a refractory, post-transplantation, large B-cell lymphoma to an anti-CD22 immunotoxin. Ann Intern Med 1997;126:882–5.

[43] Kreitman RJ, Hansen HJ, Jones AL, et al. Pseudomonas exotoxin-based immunotoxins containing the antibody LL2 or LL2-Fab' induce regression of subcutaneous human B-cell lymphoma in mice. Cancer Res 1993;53:819–25.

[44] Theuer CP, Kreitman RJ, FitzGerald DJ, et al. Immunotoxins made with a recombinant form of Pseudomonas exotoxin A that do not require proteolysis for activity. Cancer Res 1993;53:340–7.

[45] Mansfield E, Chiron MF, Amlot P, et al. Recombinant RFB4 single-chain immunotoxin that is cytotoxic towards CD22-positive cells. Biochem Soc Trans 1997;25:709–14.

[46] Mansfield E, Amlot P, Pastan I, et al. Recombinant RFB4 immunotoxins exhibit potent cytotoxic activity for CD22-bearing cells and tumors. Blood 1997;90:2020–6.

[47] Kreitman RJ, Wang QC, FitzGerald DJP, et al. Complete regression of human B-cell lymphoma xenografts in mice treated with recombinant anti-CD22 immunotoxin RFB4(dsFv)-PE38 at doses tolerated by Cynomolgus monkeys. Int J Cancer 1999;81:148–55.

[48] Kreitman RJ, Margulies I, Stetler-Stevenson M, et al. Cytotoxic activity of disulfide-stabilized recombinant immunotoxin RFB4(dsFv)-PE38 (BL22) towards fresh malignant cells from patients with B-cell leukemias. Clin Cancer Res 2000;6:1476–87.

[49] Kreitman RJ, Squires DR, Stetler-Stevenson M, et al. Phase I trial of recombinant immunotoxin RFB4(dsFv)-PE38 (BL22) in patients with B-cell malignancies. J Clin Oncol 2005;23:6719–29.

[50] Kreitman RJ, Wilson WH, Bergeron K, et al. Efficacy of the anti-CD22 recombinant immunotoxin BL22 in chemotherapy-resistant hairy-cell leukemia. N Engl J Med 2001;345:241–7.

[51] Tallman MS, Hakimian D, Kopecky KJ, et al. Minimal residual disease in patients with hairy cell leukemia in complete remission treated with 2-chlorodeoxyadenosine or 2-deoxycoformycin and prediction of early relapse. Clin Cancer Res 1999;5:1665–70.

[52] Fujimori K, Covell DG, Fletcher JE, et al. Modeling analysis of the global and microscopic distribution of immunoglobulin G, F(ab')2, and Fab in tumors. Cancer Res 1989;49:5656–63.

[53] Moake JL. Thrombotic microangiopathies. N Engl J Med 2002;347:589–600.

Hematol Oncol Clin N Am 20 (2006) 1153–1162

HEMATOLOGY/ONCOLOGY CLINICS
OF NORTH AMERICA

SEVIER
UNDERS

Hairy Cell Leukemia: Towards a Curative Strategy

Adi Gidron, MD, Martin S. Tallman, MD*

Division of Hematology/Oncology, Department of Medicine, Northwestern University Feinberg School of Medicine, 676 North St. Clair, Suite 850, Chicago IL, 60611 USA

Hairy cell leukemia (HCL) is one of the rarest of the chronic lymphoproliferative disorders, but is now among the most effectively treated. The disease usually is easy to diagnose because of the characteristic proliferation of a malignant clone of B cells with irregular cytoplasmic projections [1]. Despite the usually indolent course of HCL, most patients require therapy when cytopenias become life threatening or when they develop symptomatic splenomegaly, which, generally, is the sole physical finding. Before the introduction of purine analogs, treatment with splenectomy and interferon-α was a common approach that led to clinical and hematologic responses, but they rarely were complete and median survival was only 4 years [2,3]. Patients who undergo splenectomy have a better 5-year overall survival (OS) than those who do not; however the 5-year survival is only 55% to 60% (Table 1) [4,5]. Table 2 summarizes the 5-year OS for patients who were treated with interferon-α.

Treatment of HCL changed dramatically approximately 20 years ago when it was shown that patients who are given 2'deoxycoformycin (2'-DCF) or 2-chlorodeoxyadenosine (2-CdA) achieve durable complete remissions (CRs) [6,7]. Treatment with 2-CdA or 2'-DCF results in 80% to 90% CR with a relapse rate of 25% to 30% at 3- to 5-year follow-up [8]. In the past several years, several reports of long-term follow-up confirm excellent durability of responses. In addition, effective new therapies, such as rituximab and BL22, have been introduced.

MECHANISMS OF ACTIVITY OF PURINE ANALOGS IN HAIRY CELL LEUKEMIA

The cytotoxic effects of purine analogs are mediated by induction of DNA strand breaks and inhibition of DNA repair by impairing ribonucleotide reductase. However, the purine analogs have different specific mechanisms of action. Fludarabine and 2-CdA inhibit ribonucleotide reductase and interfere with DNA polymerase by competing with 2'-deoxyadenosine 5'triphosphate

*Corresponding author. E-mail address: m-tallman@northwestern.edu (M.S. Tallman).

0889-8588/06/$ – see front matter
doi:10.1016/j.hoc.2006.06.004

Table 1
Treatments of historical interest. Overall survival (4–5 y) following splenectomy in hairy cell leukemia

Study [Ref]	Splenectomy	No splenectomy
Flandrin et al, 1984 [5]	60%	42%
Jansen and Hermans, 1981 [45]	55%	38%

(dATP) [9]. In addition, these agents lead to DNA strand breaks and prevent repair in resting cells [10]. In contrast, 2'-DCF is an irreversible inhibitor of adenosine deaminase that leads to the accumulation of triphosphate metabolites that inhibit DNA synthesis in dividing cells [9].

LONG-TERM FOLLOW-UP OF PATIENTS WHO HAD HAIRY CELL LEUKEMIA THAT WAS TREATED WITH PURINE ANALOGS

Several long-term follow-up studies have been published recently. Chadha and colleagues [11] reported on 86 patients who were treated between 1990 and 2003 with a single 7-day course of 2-CdA by continuous infusion at a dosage of 0.1 mg/kg/d. Seventy-nine percent of patients achieved CR and 21% achieved partial response (PR). At a median follow-up of 9.7 years (range, 0.3–13.8 years), 31 (36%) patients relapsed. Twenty-three of the relapsing patients were treated with a second cycle of 2-CdA with an overall response rate (OR) of 83% (52% CR, 30% PR). The OS rate at 12 years was 87% [11]. Else and colleagues [12] reported on 219 patients with a median follow-up of 12.5 years (range, 1–34.6 years). One hundred eighty-five patients were treated with 2'-DCF and 34 patients were treated with 2-CdA as first-line therapy. Ninety-four patients did not have any previous therapy, whereas the remainder had undergone a splenectomy, received interferon-α, or both. Most patients who were treated with 2'-DCF received 4 mg/m^2 intravenously (IV) every 2 weeks until maximal response plus two consolidation cycles. Patients who received 2-CdA were treated as described above. Response, relapse rate, and OS at 10 years were similar between the treatment groups. 2'-DCF was associated with a CR rate of 81% compared with 82% for 2-CdA. The OS was 96% and 100% with 2'-DCF and 2-CdA, respectively. Although an earlier report of

Table 2
Treatments of historical interest. Overall survival (4–5 y) with interferon

Study	Overall survival (%)
Ratain et al, 1988 [46]	91
Smith et al, 1991 [47]	86
Capnist et al, 1994 [48]	85
Federico et al, 1994 [4]	96
Frassoldati et al, 1994 [49]	89
Rai et al, 1995 [50]	83

the same series found an advantage for 2'-DCF in reducing the relapse rate, the updated study did not find such a difference after longer follow-up [8]. In both studies, achieving CR was associated with better OS [11,12]. These reports, and others, indicate that both purine analogs are highly effective and lead to excellent OS (Table 3). However, it appears that neither purine analog is likely curative because molecular studies suggest that all patients have evidence of minimal residual disease (MRD) while in CR [13]. These data suggest that further therapy following purine analogs for MRD, perhaps with a potentially minimally toxic agent (eg, rituximab), may be a useful strategy to pursue.

CURRENT TREATMENT RECOMMENDATIONS
Dosing Schedules
2' Deoxycoformycin
It is now well established that purine analogs are the treatment of choice as first-line therapy in HCL. Long-term follow-up studies suggest no clear advantage for one purine analog over the other [12]. 2'-DCF usually is given at a dosage of 4 mg/m^2 by IV bolus every 2 weeks and is continued until maximal response. Maintenance therapy is unnecessary. Myelosuppression and infections are the most commonly reported toxicities, but gastrointestinal, hepatic, renal, and neurologic toxicity also are reported [9,14,15]. When higher doses were used (5 mg/m^2 on 2 consecutive days every 2 weeks), severe neutropenia was noted in 26% of patients and 6% of patients died of infections [16]. OR was 87% and was not better than with the standard schedule of 4 mg/m^2 every 2 weeks [17]. In fact, when an even smaller dosage was used (4 mg/m^2 every week for 3 weeks in a 8-week cycle), 25 of 28 patients achieved CR and 3 achieved PR. Toxicities were less in the studies with lower dosages, and most oncologists now treat with 4 mg/m^2 every 2 weeks for ease of administration [18]. Although response rates are high with either purine analog, 2'-DCF requires multiple cycles over several weeks and seems to be associated with a slightly worse toxicity profile than does 2-CdA.

2-Chlorodeoxyadenosine
2-CdA is administered commonly as a single course at a dosage of 0.1 mg/kg/d by continuous infusion for 7 days. Although OR and OS are not significantly different than those achieved with 2'-DCF, 2-CdA offers several advantages [12]. The toxicity profile of 2-CdA seems to be better than that of 2'-DCF. In a large study by Cheson and colleagues [19], 979 patients were treated with 2-CdA for HCL. Severe (grade 3–4) toxicities were noted in 28% of patients (mostly infectious), and life-threatening toxicities were reported in 6% of patients. Ten deaths were attributed to 2-CdA administration. When given at a dosage of 0.14 mg/kg/d by 2-hour infusion daily for 5 days or at a dosage of 0.14 mg/kg over 2 hours once a week for 5 weeks, OS was 100% and relapse rate at 122 months was 27% [20]. The ease of administration, the short duration of therapy, and the high response rate make 2-CdA an attractive first-line agent in HCL.

Table 3
2-chlorodeoxyadenosine and 2'deoxycoformycin in hairy cell leukemia: long-term outcomes

Study	Agent	N	Previously untreated	CR (%)	PR (%)	Median follow-up (mo)	Relapse (%)	Median time to relapse (mo)
Saven et al [24]	2-CdA	349	179	91	7	58	26	CR:30, PR:24
Jehn et al [36]	2-CdA	44	44	98	2	102	39	48
Chadha et al [11]	2-CdA	86	60	79	21	116	36	CR:35, PR 10.5
Else et al [12]	2-CdA	34	18	82	18	150	48	NA
Else et al [12]	2'-DCF	185	76	81	15	150	42	NA
Flinn et al [28]	2'-DCF	241	154	72	NA	112	18	NA
Maloisel et al [14]	2'-DCF	238	84	79	17	64	15	NA

Abbreviation: NA, not available.

LONG-TERM SEQUELAE

Treatment with purine analogs is associated with a prolonged period of immune suppression by decreasing $CD4^+$ lymphocytes [21–23]. The most common late infection is dermatomal herpes zoster [14,24]. A concern remains whether the prolonged immune suppression predisposes patients to secondary malignancies. The excess frequency of secondary malignancies was 1.88 in one series [24]. In a 2014 patient follow-up from the National Cancer Institute (NCI), a small trend toward an increased risk for second cancers was noted (observed/expected ratio of 1.43, 1.50, and 1.63 for patients who were treated with 2'-DCF, fludarabine, and 2-CdA, respectively). Despite reaching statistical significance in patients who were treated with fludarabine and 2-CdA, the incidence is consistent with the increase that already is associated with HCL [25,26]. Other studies fail to show an increased risk for secondary malignancies, although some of them noted an increased risk for lymphoid malignancies [27–29]. Given these long-term sequelae, prophylactic therapy with an antiviral agent can be considered, and close monitoring for second cancers is recommended.

MINIMAL RESIDUAL DISEASE AFTER TREATMENT WITH PURINE ANALOGS

Despite high response rates and long disease-free survival (DFS) that are associated with purine analog therapy, relapses occur in a substantial number of patients, which suggests the presence of MRD. When patients are evaluated for MRD by immunohistochemistry with stains that react with CD20, DBA 44, and anti-CD45RO, immunophenotyping by flow cytometry, or consensus polymerase chain reaction, 50% to 100% of complete responders have MRD [13,30–32]. Treatment with rituximab after 2-CdA resulted in an increase in molecular remission and lower levels of MRD than those found before rituximab treatment [33]. Despite the presence of MRD detected by molecular techniques, some studies failed to link MRD to relapse risk [34]. Although MRD may or may not be associated with shorter DFS, it is not recommended to treat MRD because not all patients have recurrence of disease, and it is not known if such an intervention improves survival [34,35].

TREATMENT OF RELAPSED DISEASE

Relapses occur in up to 40% of patients in several long-term follow-ups, regardless of the purine analog that was used as first-line therapy (Table 3) [11,12, 14,24,28,36]. After relapse, treatment with an additional course of purine analogs is recommended. It is acceptable to repeat the same treatment that was given initially, although changing to a different purine analog will yield the same results. Although the ability to attain a CR decreases with each course of therapy, the probability of achieving CR does not seem to be affected by the agent that is used [12]. When the same agent is used, CR is attained by 71% of patients compared with 68% of those who change to the alternate purine analog. The relapse rates are approximately the same after subsequent courses of therapy (35% and 28% after second and third courses, respectively), but DFS appears to be shorter after each course [12]. Of the 979 patients who were treated by Cheson and colleagues [19], 68 patients who were treated with 2′-DCF relapsed, and were retreated with 2-CdA. Seventy-nine percent achieved a CR. In other studies, response rates to second-line therapy exceed 82% [11,20,36]. A trend toward shorter DFS after second-line therapy also is observed in these studies. Although a substantial number of patients remain disease-free for a prolonged period of time, more than one third eventually relapse. Retreatment with purine analogs is associated with a high response rate; however, some patients become refractory to this class of agent.

OTHER AGENTS THAT ARE EFFECTIVE FOR THE TREATMENT OF RELAPSED DISEASE

Rituximab

Recently, monoclonal antibodies have emerged as a useful strategy for patients who have relapsed or refractory HCL. Rituximab is an anti-CD20 monoclonal antibody with activity in a variety of lymphoproliferative diseases. Rituximab appears to be useful in eradicating MRD after treatment with a purine analog [37]; however, it is not clear if this strategy leads to a survival benefit. The role of rituximab in the treatment of relapsed disease is evolving. Of patients who had relapsed disease after treatment with 2-CdA, who were treated with 375 mg/m^2 of rituximab weekly for 4 weeks, only 25% had a response (6/24 patients had a response [3 CRs and 3 PRs]) [38]. When 15 patients who had relapsed or refractory HCL were treated with 8 weekly courses of rituximab at a dosage of 375 mg/m^2, 12 patients responded, 8 of them with a CR. After a median follow-up of 32 months 5 patients progressed [39]. It is possible that longer courses or higher dosages are necessary for a better response. Larger randomized studies are lacking, but it is clear that rituximab is active in HCL, provides an easy and safe alternative for patients who have relapsed or refractory HCL, and potentially has a role in eradicating MRD (Table 4).

Table 4
Treatment of relapsed or refractory disease

Study	N	Agent	CR/PR/NR
Kreitman et al [42]	31	BL22	19/6/6
Lauria et al [51]	10	Mabthera	1/4/5
Nieva et al [38]	24	Rituximab	3/3/18
Hagberg & Lundholm [52]	11	Rituximab	6/1/4
Thomas et al [39]	15	Rituximab	8/4/3

BL22

BL22 is one of the most promising new agents for the treatment of HCL. BL22 is an anti-CD22 monoclonal antibody that is linked chemically to truncated *Pseudomonas* exotoxin A, and has excellent activity against B cells in vitro and in vivo [40]. Early-phase studies of BL22 in patients who had refractory HCL revealed marked activity of this agent. Eleven of 16 patients achieved CR in a phase I dosage-escalating study [41]. In an update of the same trial, 25 of 31 patients responded to therapy (19 CRs). Achieving a CR was associated with a greater than 90% reduction in circulating hairy cells by the third dosage. In addition, it seems that most patients with CRs did not have MRD detected in the bone marrow. Durable response (median CR duration of 36 months) was associated with faster response to therapy. In general, toxicities were mild and consisted of fatigue, myalgia, transaminitis, and hypoalbuinemia. The more serious side effects included hemolytic uremic syndrome and cytokine release syndrome with vascular leak that occurred with the 50-μg/kg dosage. Therefore, 40 μg/kg was established as the safe dose [42]. A mutant form of BL22, termed HA22, which has a greater affinity to CD22, is under development. In preclinical trials HA22 had a twofold increase in cytotoxic activity as compared with BL22 on several CD22-positive cell lines [43].

Alemtuzumab

Alemtuzumab is a humanized anti-CD52 monoclonal antibody with activity in several lymphoproliferative diseases. HCL cells express CD52 in 92% to 100% of cases [44]. It is possible that alemtuzumab will have activity, but data are lacking as to the effectiveness of alemtuzumab in the treatment of HCL.

Novel targeted therapies, such as rituximab and BL22, are active in HCL and provide minimally toxic options for patients who have relapsed or refractory disease. Dosing schedules are still under investigation and their role as first-line therapy has not been investigated.

SUMMARY

Although not all patients who have HCL require therapy at diagnosis, most eventually need treatment. Historically, splenectomy and interferon-α resulted in hematologic responses; however, responses tend to be short. The introduction of purine analogs dramatically changed the prognosis for most patients who have HCL. It is now considered standard of care to use a purine analog, such as 2-CdA or 2′-DCF, as first-line therapy. This approach results in a high CR rate and prolonged DFS. Although both agents yield the same rates of CR and survival, 2-CdA seems easier to administer and may be associated with less toxicity. Despite the excellent results with purine analogs, most patients have MRD detected by sensitive techniques; 30% to 40% of patients eventually relapse and most require further therapy. A repeat course of 2-CdA (or 2′-DCF) will result in CR in approximately 70% of patients. For patients who have relapsed or refractory disease, monoclonal antibody–based therapies are emerging options. Rituximab and BL22 are highly active in this setting. Until BL22 becomes widely available, rituximab is a reasonable choice for salvage

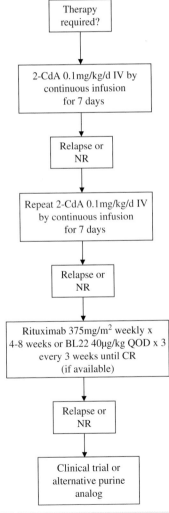

Fig. 1. A suggested algorithm for the treatment of hairy cell leukemia. QOD, every other day.

therapy; however, the dosing schedule needs to be defined further. The roles of rituximab and BL22 as initial therapy for patients who have previously untreated HCL have not been investigated. Fig. 1 is a suggested algorithm for the treatment of HCL. With the introduction of effective new agents, further studies will determine whether the now achievable prolonged survival will translate into cure.

References

[1] Golomb HM, Catovsky D, Golde DW. Hairy cell leukemia: a clinical review based on 71 cases. Ann Intern Med 1978;89(5 Pt 1):677–83.

[2] Berman E, Heller G, Kempin S, et al. Incidence of response and long-term follow-up in patients with hairy cell leukemia treated with recombinant interferon alfa-2a. Blood 1990; 75(4):839–45.

[3] Grever M, Kopecky K, Foucar MK, et al. Randomized comparison of pentostatin versus interferon alfa-2a in previously untreated patients with hairy cell leukemia: an intergroup study. J Clin Oncol 1995;13(4):974–82.

[4] Federico M, Frassoldati A, Lamparelli T, et al. Long-term results of alpha interferon as initial therapy and splenectomy as consolidation therapy in patients with hairy cell leukemia. Final report from the Italian Cooperative Group for HCL. Ann Oncol 1994;5(8):725–31.

[5] Flandrin G, Sigaux F, Sebahoun G, et al. Hairy cell leukemia: clinical presentation and follow-up of 211 patients. Semin Oncol 1984; 11 (4) (Suppl 2):458–71.

[6] Spiers AS, Moore D, Cassileth PA, et al. Remissions in hairy-cell leukemia with pentostatin (2'-deoxycoformycin). N Engl J Med 1987;316(14):825–30.

[7] Piro LD, Carrera CJ, Carson DA, et al. Lasting remissions in hairy-cell leukemia induced by a single infusion of 2-chlorodeoxyadenosine. N Engl J Med 1990;322(16):1117–21.

[8] Dearden CE, Matutes E, Hilditch BL, et al. Long-term follow-up of patients with hairy cell leukaemia after treatment with pentostatin or cladribine. Br J Haematol 1999;106(2): 515–9.

[9] Tallman MS, Hakimian D. Purine nucleoside analogs: emerging roles in indolent lymphoproliferative disorders. Blood 1995;86(7):2463–74.

[10] Seto S, Carrera CJ, Kubota M, et al. Mechanism of deoxyadenosine and 2-chlorodeoxyadenosine toxicity to nondividing human lymphocytes. J Clin Invest 1985;75(2):377–83.

[11] Chadha P, Rademaker AW, Mendiratta P, et al. Treatment of hairy cell leukemia with 2-chlorodeoxyadenosine (2-CdA): long-term follow-up of the Northwestern University experience. Blood 2005;106(1):241–6.

[12] Else M, Ruchlemer R, Osuji N, et al. Long remissions in hairy cell leukemia with purine analogs: a report of 219 patients with a median follow-up of 12.5 years. Cancer 2005; 104(11):2442–8.

[13] Filleul B, Delannoy A, Ferrant A, et al. A single course of 2-chlorodeoxyadenosine does not eradicate leukemic cells in hairy cell leukemia patients in complete remission. Leukemia 1994;8(7):1153–6.

[14] Maloisel F, Benboubker L, Gardembas M, et al. Long-term outcome with pentostatin treatment in hairy cell leukemia patients. A French retrospective study of 238 patients. Leukemia 2003;17(1):45–51.

[15] Rafel M, Cervantes F, Beltran JM, et al. Deoxycoformycin in the treatment of patients with hairy cell leukemia: results of a Spanish collaborative study of 80 patients. Cancer 2000; 88(2):352–7.

[16] Cassileth PA, Cheuvart B, Spiers AS, et al. Pentostatin induces durable remissions in hairy cell leukemia. J Clin Oncol 1991;9(2):243–6.

[17] Kraut EH, Bouroncle BA, Grever MR. Pentostatin in the treatment of advanced hairy cell leukemia. J Clin Oncol 1989;7(2):168–72.

[18] Johnston JB, Eisenhauer E, Corbett WE, et al. Efficacy of 2'-deoxycoformycin in hairy-cell leukemia: a study of the National Cancer Institute of Canada Clinical Trials Group. J Natl Cancer Inst 1988;80(10):765–9.

[19] Cheson BD, Sorensen JM, Vena DA, et al. Treatment of hairy cell leukemia with 2-chlorodeoxyadenosine via the Group C protocol mechanism of the National Cancer Institute: a report of 979 patients. J Clin Oncol 1998;16(9):3007–15.

[20] Zinzani PL, Tani M, Marchi E, et al. Long-term follow-up of front-line treatment of hairy cell leukemia with 2-chlorodeoxyadenosine. Haematologica 2004;89(3):309–13.

[21] Seymour JF, Kurzrock R, Freireich EJ, et al. 2-chlorodeoxyadenosine induces durable remissions and prolonged suppression of CD4$^+$ lymphocyte counts in patients with hairy cell leukemia. Blood 1994;83(10):2906–11.

[22] Seymour JF, Talpaz M, Kurzrock R. Response duration and recovery of CD4$^+$ lymphocytes following deoxycoformycin in interferon-alpha-resistant hairy cell leukemia: 7-year follow-up. Leukemia 1997;11(1):42–7.

[23] Urba WJ, Baseler MW, Kopp WC, et al. Deoxycoformycin-induced immunosuppression in patients with hairy cell leukemia. Blood 1989;73(1):38–46.

[24] Saven A, Burian C, Koziol JA, et al. Long-term follow-up of patients with hairy cell leukemia after cladribine treatment. Blood 1998;92(6):1918–26.

[25] Au WY, Klasa RJ, Gallagher R, et al. Second malignancies in patients with hairy cell leukemia in British Columbia: a 20-year experience. Blood 1998;92(4):1160–4.

[26] Cheson BD, Vena DA, Barrett J, et al. Second malignancies as a consequence of nucleoside analog therapy for chronic lymphoid leukemias. J Clin Oncol 1999;17(8):2454–60.

[27] Federico M, Zinzani PL, Frassoldati A, et al. Risk of second cancer in patients with hairy cell leukemia: long-term follow-up. J Clin Oncol 2002;20(3):638–46.

[28] Flinn IW, Kopecky KJ, Foucar MK, et al. Long-term follow-up of remission duration, mortality, and second malignancies in hairy cell leukemia patients treated with pentostatin. Blood 2000;96(9):2981–6.

[29] Kurzrock R, Strom SS, Estey E, et al. Second cancer risk in hairy cell leukemia: analysis of 350 patients. J Clin Oncol 1997;15(5):1803–10.

[30] Ellison DJ, Sharpe RW, Robbins BA, et al. Immunomorphologic analysis of bone marrow biopsies after treatment with 2-chlorodeoxyadenosine for hairy cell leukemia. Blood 1994;84(12):4310–5.

[31] Sausville JE, Salloum RG, Sorbara L, et al. Minimal residual disease detection in hairy cell leukemia. Comparison of flow cytometric immunophenotyping with clonal analysis using consensus primer polymerase chain reaction for the heavy chain gene. Am J Clin Pathol 2003;119(2):213–7.

[32] Wheaton S, Tallman MS, Hakimian D, et al. Minimal residual disease may predict bone marrow relapse in patients with hairy cell leukemia treated with 2-chlorodeoxyadenosine. Blood 1996;87(4):1556–60.

[33] Cervetti G, Galimberti S, Andreazzoli F, et al. Rituximab as treatment for minimal residual disease in hairy cell leukaemia. Eur J Haematol 2004;73(6):412–7.

[34] Matutes E, Meeus P, McLennan K, et al. The significance of minimal residual disease in hairy cell leukaemia treated with deoxycoformycin: a long-term follow-up study. Br J Haematol 1997;98(2):375–83.

[35] Tallman MS, Hakimian D, Kopecky KJ, et al. Minimal residual disease in patients with hairy cell leukemia in complete remission treated with 2-chlorodeoxyadenosine or 2-deoxycoformycin and prediction of early relapse. Clin Cancer Res 1999;5(7):1665–70.

[36] Jehn U, Bartl R, Dietzfelbinger H, et al. An update: 12-year follow-up of patients with hairy cell leukemia following treatment with 2-chlorodeoxyadenosine. Leukemia 2004;18(9):1476–81.

[37] Farhad Ravandi-Kashani SOB, Keating M, Jones D, et al. Complete eradication of minimal residual disease (MRD) in patients with hairy cell leukemia (HCL), after cladribine (2CDA) followed by an extended course of rituximab. [abstract]. Blood 2005;106(11):911a.

[38] Nieva J, Bethel K, Saven A. Phase 2 study of rituximab in the treatment of cladribine-failed patients with hairy cell leukemia. Blood 2003;102(3):810–3.

[39] Thomas DA, O'Brien S, Bueso-Ramos C, et al. Rituximab in relapsed or refractory hairy cell leukemia. Blood 2003;102(12):3906–11.

[40] Kreitman RJ, Wilson WH, Robbins D, et al. Responses in refractory hairy cell leukemia to a recombinant immunotoxin. Blood 1999;94(10):3340–8.

[41] Kreitman RJ, Wilson WH, Bergeron K, et al. Efficacy of the anti-CD22 recombinant immunotoxin BL22 in chemotherapy-resistant hairy-cell leukemia. N Engl J Med 2001;345(4): 241–7.

[42] Kreitman RJ, Squires DR, Stetler-Stevenson M, et al. Phase I trial of recombinant immunotoxin RFB4(dsFv)-PE38 (BL22) in patients with B-cell malignancies. J Clin Oncol 2005;23(27): 6719–29.

[43] Bang S, Nagata S, Onda M, et al. HA22 (R490A) is a recombinant immunotoxin with increased antitumor activity without an increase in animal toxicity. Clin Cancer Res 2005; 11(4):1545–50.

[44] Quigley MM, Bethel KJ, Sharpe RW, et al. CD52 expression in hairy cell leukemia. Am J Hematol 2003;74(4):227–30.

[45] Jansen J, Hermans J. Splenectomy in hairy cell leukemia: a retrospective multicenter analysis. Cancer 1981;47(8):2066–76.

[46] Ratain MJ, Golomb HM, Vardiman JW, et al. Relapse after interferon alfa-2b therapy for hairy-cell leukemia: analysis of prognostic variables. J Clin Oncol 1988;6(11):1714–21.

[47] Smith JW II, Longo DL, Urba WJ, et al. Prolonged, continuous treatment of hairy cell leukemia patients with recombinant interferon-alpha 2a. Blood 1991;78(7):1664–71.

[48] Capnist G, Federico M, Chisesi T, et al. Long term results of interferon treatment in hairy cell leukemia. Italian Cooperative Group of Hairy Cell Leukemia (ICGHCL). Leuk Lymphoma 1994;14(5–6):457–64.

[49] Frassoldati A, Lamparelli T, Federico M, et al. Hairy cell leukemia: a clinical review based on 725 cases of the Italian Cooperative Group (ICGHCL). Italian Cooperative Group for Hairy Cell Leukemia. Leuk Lymphoma 1994;13(3–4):307–16.

[50] Rai KR, Davey F, Peterson B, et al. Recombinant alpha-2b-interferon in therapy of previously untreated hairy cell leukemia: long-term follow-up results of study by Cancer and Leukemia Group B. Leukemia 1995;9(7):1116–20.

[51] Lauria F, Lenoci M, Annino L, et al. Efficacy of anti-CD20 monoclonal antibodies (Mabthera) in patients with progressed hairy cell leukemia. Haematologica 2001;86(10):1046–50.

[52] Hagberg H, Lundholm L. Rituximab, a chimaeric anti-CD20 monoclonal antibody, in the treatment of hairy cell leukaemia. Br J Haematol 2001;115(3):609–11.

HEMATOLOGY/ONCOLOGY CLINICS
OF NORTH AMERICA

INDEX

Note: Page numbers of article titles are in **boldface** type.

0889-8588/06/$ – see front matter
doi:10.1016/S0889-8588(06)00144-4